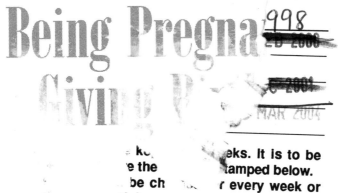

Being Pregna

Giving

ks.   eeks. It is to be
e the   tamped below.
be ch   every week or
k is ove   ue.

Being Pregnant Giving Birth

Mary Nolan

A
NATIONAL CHILDBIRTH TRUST
GUIDE

Published by National Childbirth Trust Publishing
in collaboration with Thorsons

Thorsons
An Imprint of HarperCollins*Publishers*

Picture Acknowledgements

The publishers would like to thank the following for their permission to
reproduce photographs: Tony Stone Images/Nigel Hillier: Cover;
Ian Keys: pxiv; The Image Bank/Romilly Lockyer: p30; MIDIRS: pp42, 92, 116;
Lupe Cunha Photography: pp66, 148; Michael Bassett: p170; Eddie Lawrence: p184.

Illustrations: Jo Dennis, Pete Welford.

Design by Tim McPhee.

Production in association with
Book Production Consultants plc,
25–27 High Street, Chesterton, Cambridge CB4 1ND, UK.

Printed by Hillman Printers (Frome) Ltd,
Frome, Somerset.

Published by National Childbirth Trust Publishing,
25-27 High Street, Chesterton, Cambridge CB4 1ND, UK.

in collaboration with Thorsons
An Imprint of HarperCollins *Publishers*
77–85 Fulham Palace Road, Hammersmith, London W6 8JB.

© 1996 NCT Publishing

First published 1996
This edition 1998

A CIP catalogue record for this book is available from the British Library.

ISBN 0 7225 3636 4

Contents

About the author

MARY NOLAN trained as an antenatal teacher with The National Childbirth Trust from 1985–1987. Since then, she has prepared many women and couples for birth and parenthood, and has worked with young people in schools, exploring with them what is involved in having a baby and attempting to minimise the fear of childbirth which is endemic in our culture. Mary has talked to student nurses and midwives about the needs of women during pregnancy, in labour and after the birth of their babies and has organised many workshops to help health professionals gain deeper insight into the support they can offer to women and their families during the childbearing year. Recently, she has become known as an author on birth issues, with articles appearing in the midwifery and popular press. Mary lives in Worcestershire with her partner, Peter, and three young daughters.

Contributors

BARBARA KOTT is president of the NCT and has 18 years' experience working with the Trust as an antenatal teacher and tutor. During that time she has worked with midwives and health professionals, and has been involved in training other antenatal teachers and tutors throughout Europe.

PAULINE ARMSTRONG is a sociologist and has worked as an antenatal teacher and tutor for the Trust for 15 years. She too has many years' experience of working with midwives and health professionals. She is an ex-executive of MIDIRS (Midwives Information and Resource Service) where she was involved in medical research.

Publisher's note

ALL COMMENTS and personal accounts were given to us in confidence, so out of respect for our contributors' privacy we have omitted their names.

We have endeavoured where possible to reproduce quotations verbatim, but where editing has been applied, the integrity of the quotation has been maintained.

Acknowledgements

THIS BOOK REPRESENTS the combined efforts of a lot of people. Firstly, I would like to thank all those antenatal tutors from The National Childbirth Trust who organised focus groups so that women could talk about their pregnancies and labours, share their fears and joys, and get support and comfort from each other. I cannot praise sufficiently the courage and insight shown by the women who participated in these groups and their generosity in allowing their thoughts and feelings to be quoted in bringing this book to life. I also want to thank my own antenatal teacher; students who commented on various aspects of the book, provided me with new material, and were generally enthusiastic and encouraging. Certain individuals deserve special mention for their magnificent help and these are Elisabeth Buggins, Nikki Ford, Judy Letters, Wendy Mockridge, Morven Lawson, Vicky Baughen and NCT's two librarians, Patricia Donnithorne and Eileen Abbott. Thank you finally to my family, Peter, Sophie, Roisin and Alexandra, who put up with my short temper in the days running up to the deadline for this book to be finished!

The tutors who did the research for the book are: Jeanne Langford, Val Humphreys, Nina Smith, Anna Louise Sheppherd, Jill Davidson, Margaret Short, Debbie Garrod and Elisabeth Buggins.

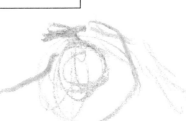

Introduction

THE DAY ON which your baby is born is probably going to be one of the most important days of your life. It is an amazing experience to bring a new person into the world – an experience that will make tremendous demands on you both physically and emotionally. The things that happen to you when you give birth will stay with you for the rest of your life and may influence the way in which you mother your child.

Today, the health services recognise that people feel more satisfied with their care and are less likely to complain if professionals ask them what kind of care they want. In one way, the new approach is very liberating, but it certainly puts a burden of responsibility upon us to gather information, look at the options available, and then make considered choices. This can be a little frightening, but it's also exciting because it means that you can shape your pregnancy care to suit your own needs, and plan for a labour that will make the birth of your baby an experience you can look back on with satisfaction.

Doctors and midwives are experts about pregnancy, labour and new babies, but they are not experts about you. What you want and need, what will make you feel most content in labour and after your baby is born, will be different from what any other woman wants and needs. You are the expert about you. Of course, you will want to listen to the professional advice of your midwife and doctor, but then you can consider how what they have said fits in with your own understanding of what will suit you best. Making choices does not mean that you are setting yourself up against health professionals, but rather that you are working in partnership with them to achieve the best outcome for you and your baby.

There are many things which you can make a choice about when you are pregnant, during your labour and after the birth of your baby. Some women choose not to make any choices. They feel that they will be happiest if health professionals make all their decisions for them and prefer to hand over control to midwives and doctors. This is one kind of choice.

However, other women want to keep control over what is happening to them; they feel frightened and belittled if health professionals decide what to do without consulting them. Women who consider that having a baby is a normal, everyday event and who sense that they know more about themselves and their unborn babies than anyone else feel that they have the right and the responsibility to participate in their own care and to be part of the decision-making team.

The maternity services, like all big organisations, can often seem to be a conveyor belt to the women using them. However, very often, it is simply necessary to speak out and *ask* for what you want and staff will suddenly turn out to be far more accommodating than you had imagined them:

'Once we'd explained that we didn't want to be railroaded, I found the staff in hospital extremely supportive, coming up with ideas before I could think of them myself. I've found going there a very positive experience.'

GETTING INFORMATION about different kinds of maternity care and learning about what will happen to you when you give birth to your baby are wonderful confidence boosters. There is great satisfaction to be had from knowing that you are in a good position to make decisions about your own care during pregnancy and labour because you are well informed:

'When there are choices to be made, at least I'll be well informed. I hope things go according to plan, but even if they don't, I still feel confident that I'll cope better than if I'd not tried to find out as much as I can.'

THIS BOOK AIMS to give you some of the factual information you need to make choices. It also aims to give you an idea of what having a baby and being a new mother *feel* like because choices are not made on the basis of head-logic only; they're also made according to your *instinctive* understanding of what will be best for you. The book is therefore a balance between the boxes which tell you the facts and the main body of the text which tells you how women experience the facts. It doesn't tell you what choices to make. Your choices are yours alone.

Mary Nolan
December 1995.

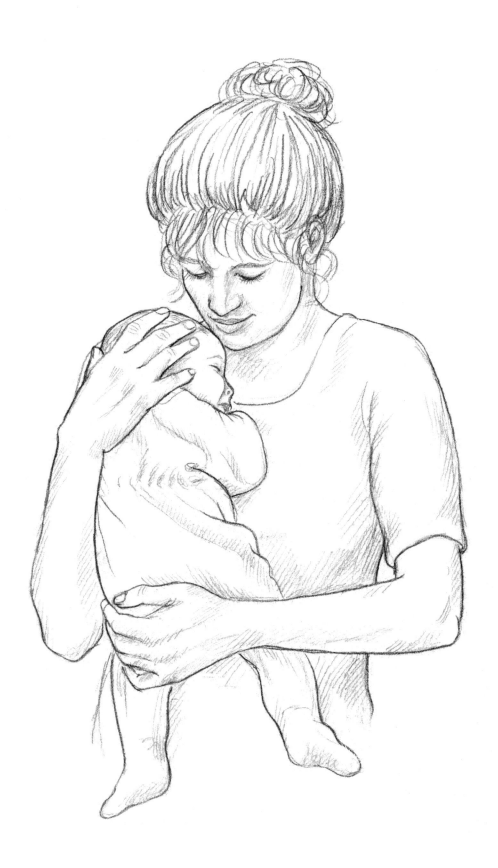

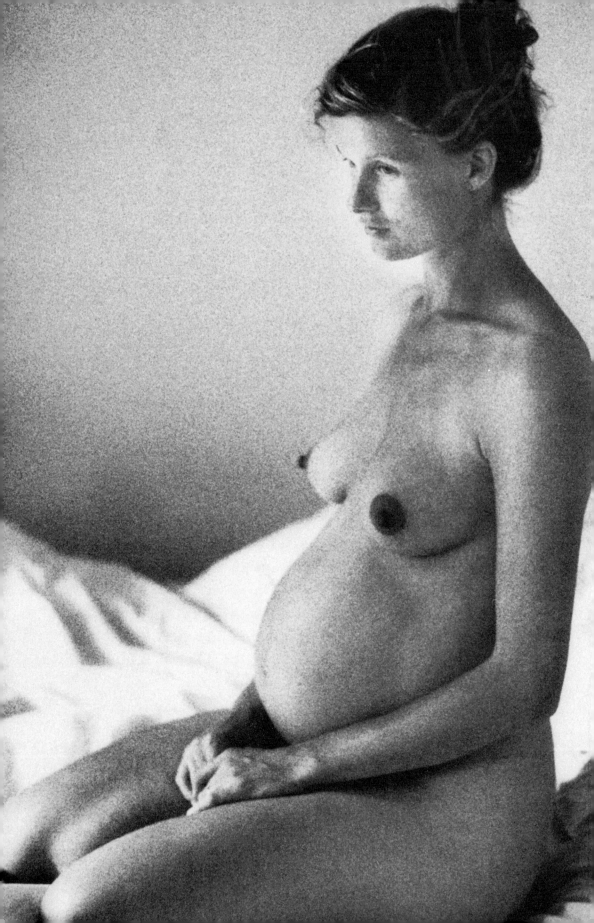

CHAPTER _one_ Pregnancy

FINDING OUT

FOR MANY WOMEN, the moment when they find out that they are pregnant for the first time is the most exciting moment of their lives:

'Deep down I had desperately wanted to have a baby and suddenly – there I was, pregnant!'

'I was ecstatic and happy and frightened, and I thought how typical it was that Duncan wasn't there to tell!'

'I was told I was expecting twins when I was eight weeks pregnant and the scan showed two hearts beating. My partner was over the moon and we immediately started speculating on what sex they would be!'

THE NEW MOTHER has a vision of all the changes and excitement of the next nine months: growing bigger and the baby's first fluttering moves inside her; being the centre of attention at family gatherings, at work and with friends; going into labour and the drama of giving birth; holding her baby in her arms for the first time and showing him off to her own mother and father and everyone she knows.

For some women, however, discovering that they are pregnant is a surprise of a different kind and doesn't provoke a sense of overwhelming joy. The pregnancy may not be wanted at this time, or not at all, and adjusting to the situation is a gradual process: _'I had mixed feelings after I found out I was pregnant. I started thinking, "Oh my God, what have we done!" My husband wanted to tell everyone immediately, but I wanted to keep the whole thing quiet until I'd got used to it.'_

YOUR 'BOOKING VISIT' OR EARLY PREGNANCY ASSESSMENT CLINIC

Shortly after your pregnancy has been confirmed by your GP, you will be invited to go to your local hospital or surgery to talk about your health and medical history and to have some tests. Alternatively, your midwife may come and see you in your own home. Many women prefer this because they feel more relaxed.

The midwife will ask you about:

- Your general health
- Your diet
- How much exercise you take
- Whether you smoke
- Whether you drink alcohol
- Whether you use any street drugs
- Whether you take any drugs prescribed by your doctor
- What kind of contraceptives you have used
- Your periods – how regular they are and when you had your last one
- Previous pregnancies and births, including abortions
- Your medical history – what illnesses you have had; whether you have had any operations; whether you suffer from asthma or epilepsy etc
- Whether members of your close family suffer from certain diseases
- Whether any members of your family are mentally or physically disabled.

Tests you will have:

- Your height may be measured
- You will be weighed
- Your blood pressure will be taken
- You will be asked to give a sample of urine so that it can be tested for blood, sugar and protein.

- You will have some blood taken:
  - to find out what blood group you are
  - to see what your haemoglobin level is (ie are you anaemic?)
  - to find out whether you are Rhesus positive or negative
  - to test for syphilis (sexually transmitted disease)
  - to find out whether you are immune to rubella
  - to test for sickle-cell disease if you are of African or West-Indian origin and thalassaemia if you are of Mediterranean, African, Middle or Far Eastern origin.

Examinations:

- The midwife or doctor will feel your tummy and may do a vaginal examination (an 'internal')
- The doctor may listen to your heart and lungs.

Finally:

- DON'T BE AFRAID TO ASK ANY QUESTIONS YOU WANT TO ASK

Use this opportunity to put your mind at rest about anything that is worrying you and to get all the information you need. It can be helpful to draw up a list of the things you want to ask before you go to your booking clinic or see your midwife so that nothing slips your mind.

'I was panic-stricken because it was completely unexpected. I had been told I probably wouldn't have children without some help and we had just a few months before we started thinking about whether we ought to be on a waiting list for IVF. But we thought we'd move house first and have a good holiday, and I remember telling Colin and he just sat there and said, "Well, what are we going to do now?"'

'Everything we'd planned for the next few years was turned upside down. It took me a long time to get used to the idea; I was walking around shell-shocked.'

This state of shock may persist for several months into the pregnancy: *'I didn't feel anything when I saw the first scan at 14 weeks. I just thought, "Right, well there's a baby." I didn't feel elated or anything at all.'*

How a woman feels about her pregnancy – happy and confident, happy but insecure, very unhappy – may influence how soon she wants other people to know about it. Some women choose to spread the news of the forthcoming baby straight away, although they had not originally intended an immediate announcement: *'I always used to think I'd keep it quiet for the first twelve weeks, but when it happened, I just wanted to tell everyone the minute I got that positive test.'*

Others decide not to spread the news until the pregnancy is well established so that if the baby does miscarry, no one need be told. It's not easy, however, to be feeling perhaps sick and almost certainly very tired, and not to be able to explain to people the reason: *'It's difficult not telling anyone for the first twelve weeks because that's when you're at your most vulnerable and when you need most support and when you want time off work because you're so tired.'*

Telling your mother can be very special. Your relationship with her will change now that you are taking the title of 'mother' yourself. As far as she is concerned, you are still her daughter, but as the mother of her grandchild, you have become something else, a woman about to take up all the challenges and live through all the hopes and fears which she herself has already experienced perhaps several times over: *'Ralph and I went home for Christmas and as soon as we were sitting down with my parents, I said, "I've got something to tell you", and my mother just*

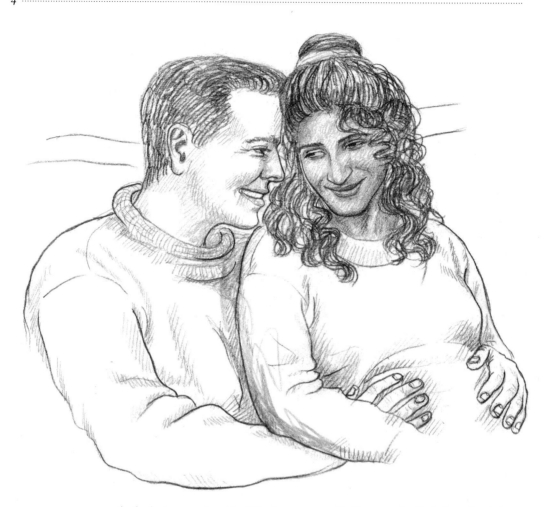

looked at me and said, "You're pregnant!" She was thrilled, but she did say to me later that it was funny knowing there were now two *generations younger than herself.'*

Anxiety during pregnancy

EVEN WHEN a baby is very much wanted, pregnancy is a time when women experience a whole variety of emotions, one of the most prominent of which is anxiety. Women who have had problems in conceiving a baby may be extremely anxious about whether they will be able to hold on to this pregnancy; women who have had previous miscarriages are fearful until they are well beyond the latest date at which they previously lost a baby; women who have given birth to a baby who afterwards died or who was disabled can spend nine months in a strained state of wondering whether the same thing might happen again: *'I was frightened all the time because I'd had several miscarriages and I was very worried about whether I was going to have another miscarriage, so the pregnancy caused mixed reactions in me.'*

'The anxiety was very strong for the first three months because I knew that this was when most IVF babies miscarried. It was less after that, but it's never really gone away. Josh and I have had this sort of nagging guilt that we weren't meant to have a baby and that because we've used technology in order to have one, we'll probably fail.'

'I haven't been as happy and excited about being pregnant as I could have been because I can't imagine how I'm going to cope with twins, and even though I've tried not to let the thought of after the birth bother me, it has.'

'Brioney died a month after she was born with heart defects. My next pregnancy was incredibly worrying as I had no confidence at all in having a healthy outcome.'

Some women really enjoy being pregnant and sail through with no problems; others are surprised by how heightened their emotions are and how the sense of responsibility is overwhelming: *'I'm not sure that I have enjoyed being pregnant; I mean I'm really looking forward to having a baby, but I've been constantly aware of everything I've eaten and everything I've done for the last eight months. I've felt very aware that it's not just me I'm affecting, it's the baby as well – a massive responsibility. If it goes wrong, I'll feel it was my fault.'*

'I always used to be a placid person. But when I became pregnant, anything I saw or heard about human suffering, especially that of children, made me immediately very emotional. I've wept buckets over reports of wars and famines.'

Your outlook on life changes and ordinary everyday activities take on a new importance: *'When I was pregnant, I remember thinking that I had to take care. If I had an accident crossing the road, it wouldn't just be me who got hurt. In a crowd of people, I wanted plenty of space – for the two of us.'*

THINGS THAT MIGHT WORRY YOU DURING PREGNANCY

The Golden Rule is:

If you are worried that something is wrong with your baby or yourself, contact your midwife, your doctor or the hospital straight away. Don't be frightened that you might be over-reacting; it's really important that you understand what is happening and are reassured.

The problem	Questions to ask yourself so that you can give useful information to the midwife or doctor	Possible explanations What to do
Bleeding during pregnancy	When did the bleeding start? How much blood are you losing? (just spots of blood, or a lot of blood like having a period?) Do you have pains in your abdomen?	Sometimes a miscarriage starts with a small amount of dark red bleeding and tummy cramps. However, during early pregnancy, it is not uncommon to have 'spotting' which means losing very small amounts of blood especially at the times when you would normally have had a period. Call your doctor or midwife and go to bed and rest until he or she visits. Is there someone you could ask to be with you?
Sickness	Is this sickness different from morning sickness? Can you think of anything you may have eaten which could have upset you? Do you feel feverish and generally unwell? Any pains in your abdomen?	Women get minor illnesses such as coughs, colds and stomach upsets during pregnancy as at any other time in their lives. However, if you think that your sickness may be due to something out of the ordinary, and certainly if you have any abdominal pain, go to see your doctor and ask for his or her advice. If you don't feel well enough to go to the surgery, telephone and ask for advice or request a home visit. Don't be put off if the receptionist isn't very helpful – be clear that you want to speak to or see the doctor or midwife. This is your body and your baby that you are worried about!
A fall	Did you hit your stomach or head when you fell? How do you feel now? Can you still feel the baby moving? (if the fall occurred after the time you first felt your baby moving)	A fall during pregnancy can be worrying. If you're not too bruised and your head is clear and you can feel your baby moving, there's probably nothing to worry about. But if you are worried, or you have any pain or concussion, or your baby doesn't seem to be moving as much as he was before, don't hesitate to call your doctor. And, if at all possible, get someone to come and look after you.

THINGS THAT MIGHT WORRY YOU DURING PREGNANCY

Severe headaches	Do you normally get headaches? Have you got spots before your eyes? Does your vision seem to be affected by your headache? Have you got pains in the top half of your abdomen?	Pregnancy is definitely stressful. You may find that you suffer from tension headaches and need to make time to relax, enjoy a bath, go out with your partner or friends, or treat yourself. Sometimes very bad headaches may be a symptom of a disease of pregnancy called Pregnancy Induced Hypertension (PIH) or pre-eclampsia. If you have spots before your eyes and pain in the upper part of your abdomen, you should call your doctor or midwife immediately.
Baby not moving as much/not moving at all	Has today been busy and you have simply not noticed your baby moving? Have you noticed a gradual decrease in your baby's movements over a few days? How long is it since you last felt your baby move?	It's not uncommon for busy women to get to the end of the day and suddenly become anxious that they haven't felt their baby move since morning. Sit down or lie down and relax for an hour and see if your baby starts moving. If you are at all anxious and feel that there's been a definite change in the pattern of your baby's movements, call your doctor, midwife or the hospital and seek advice.
Waters break (the bag of waters surrounding your baby either starts to leak or bursts with a gush of water down your legs.)	If the waters broke with a gush, how much was there and at what time did they break? If the waters are trickling out, when did you first notice any wetness, or feel that you had lost some fluid other than urine into the toilet? What colour is the fluid you are losing? Does it smell?	Sometimes a woman loses a small amount of the water in the womb and then the leak in the bag of waters appears to seal itself and nothing further happens. Often, however, losing water from around the baby means that labour is likely to start soon and your baby is going to be born. If you are less than 37 weeks pregnant, you need to contact the hospital straight away and you will be asked to go in. If you are more than 37 weeks pregnant, you should still contact your midwife or the hospital and take advice.

'The bigger I get, the more aware I become. A young chap pulled out in his car right in front of me and I had to slam the brakes on to miss him. Normally, if I wasn't pregnant, I'd have been out of the car ranting and raving at him, but I just sat still and then drove straight to my husband's work. I walked into the office and cried my eyes out. I was so frightened. I was thinking about this – the bump – not me.'

PREGNANT WOMEN are bombarded with information from health professionals and through the media regarding what they should and should not do during pregnancy – advice on smoking, drinking, eating, exercise, resting, taking drugs. Some women are able to rationalise the advice they are given and feel confident enough to reach their own conclusions: *'I haven't worried about diet, alcohol – that sort of thing very much, because I think that's just going over the top really. To be honest, I've eaten blue cheese and I've understood that small amounts of alcohol don't do any harm. I haven't pressured myself about that sort of thing.'*

'It's very important that you are happy within yourself and if having the odd glass of lager is going to help you relax, that's far more important.'

On the other hand many women become over-sensitive, anxious and distressed: *'Pregnancy does make you feel very, very guilty all the time – even just having a small glass of wine. I think I put the pressures on myself. I do something and then I think, "Oh, you shouldn't have done that" because of the baby.'*

Under these circumstances, it is quite natural that women may need constant reassurance during their pregnancies that their babies are okay: *'I have had times when I've felt very worried. When I was 16 weeks, I thought I should have felt the baby kick by now and the midwife came and listened to the heartbeat and put my mind at rest. So it's been the least little thing which has triggered me off into a bit of a panic.'*

A new self-image

DESPITE ALL the discomforts and anxiety of pregnancy, many women nonetheless feel very positive and proud at this time and enjoy the

ACHES AND PAINS IN PREGNANCY

Pregnancy brings with it so many changes in a woman's body that it is not surprising some aches and pains result. Although health professionals often describe these as 'minor disorders of pregnancy', they certainly do not seem very minor to the woman who is suffering from them! If you have a problem during your pregnancy, you should take advice from your doctor or midwife. What follows is a list of remedies that women have tried over the years for various pregnancy complaints and found helpful; some are not included in the textbooks, but textbooks don't always reflect the real experience of women! These remedies are not guaranteed to work for everyone, but it may be worth a try to see if some of them work for you.

Breast Pain

One of the earliest signs of pregnancy is very tender breasts which are painful to all but the lightest touch. Try:

- Applying hot or cold flannels gently to your breasts; putting bags of cold peas on your breasts can also help with the pain and tingling!
- Taking plenty of hot baths or showers
- Massaging your breasts gently
- Avoiding coffee and other drinks containing caffeine
- Wearing a bra in bed at night.

Carpal Tunnel Syndrome

During pregnancy, a woman's body accumulates a lot of extra fluid; some of this fluid can cause pressure on the nerves which pass through the wrists to the hands and the woman finds that she wakes up in the morning with pins and needles in her fingers. Holding a pen or a telephone for even a short period can be very uncomfortable. Most women find that their Carpal Tunnel Syndrome disappears a few weeks after the birth of their baby. Try:

- Swinging your arms vigorously for a few minutes first thing in the morning
- Keeping your hands raised as much as possible during the day
- Avoiding writing, using a keyboard or being on the telephone for any length of time
- Putting your hands in a basin of hot or cold water
- If you really can't stand the discomfort, ask your doctor about having splints.

Constipation

The hormones of pregnancy make the bowels sluggish and constipation is common; it can cause lethargy and headaches. Sometimes pregnant women are prescribed iron tablets because they are anaemic, and the tablets make the constipation worse. It may not be necessary to continue taking them (research suggests that the vast majority of women don't need iron tablets during pregnancy and that taking them if you don't need them may be harmful) or your doctor can prescribe a different brand. There are many.

Try the following:

- Drink lots of water
- Eat plenty of fibre-rich foods such as wholemeal bread, bran-based cereals, potatoes in their jackets, brown rice
- Eat five helpings of fruit and/or vegetables daily
- Eat prunes – they are an excellent laxative!
- Avoid eggs
- Drink lots of pure fruit juice
- Relax and take your time when trying to open your bowels
- Take lots of exercise.

ACHES AND PAINS IN PREGNANCY

Cramp

Pregnant women often get cramp in their legs, especially when they are in bed at night.

- Have a cup of hot/cold milk before settling for the night
- Circle your ankles and pull your toes up towards the ceiling for several minutes before getting into bed
- Put something under the bottom end of your mattress so that your legs are slightly raised. This will help your blood circulate around your feet and back up your legs during the night
- If a cramp attacks you, flex your foot vigorously upwards, and massage firmly between your first and second toes. If your partner will give you a massage, so much the better!

Heartburn

Pregnancy hormones make the valve at the top of your stomach slack. This means that acid from your stomach can escape into your gullet where it causes a burning sensation. Some women find heartburn the worst aspect of their pregnancy but it does stop when the baby is born.

- Have small, frequent meals
- Eat ginger biscuits but avoid spicy foods or those with a high fat content such as cheese, butter, cream, fatty meat and oily fish
- Drink peppermint tea, milk, ginger ale, sips of boiled water
- Avoid coffee and drinks containing caffeine (such as cola)

- Sleep propped up on a big pile of pillows. ('V' shaped pillows are excellent for preventing you from slipping down the bed while pregnant and are good for support later when you are feeding your baby.)
- Avoid bending over, especially after a meal; squat down to pick things up from the floor. Gardening may be best delayed until after your baby is born
- Your doctor can prescribe antacids which many women find helpful.

Morning Sickness

Many women find that the term 'morning' sickness is entirely inappropriate as they feel sick at all times of the day and night. It is a miserable feeling, but generally clears up after about fourteen weeks of pregnancy when the placenta starts producing the hormones which the ovaries have been responsible for until then. Sadly, some women find their sickness continues right through their pregnancies and is only cured by giving birth.

- Eat ginger biscuits, dry toast and anything containing peppermint
- Have small, frequent, starchy snacks such as bread rolls
- Eat regularly even if you don't feel like it
- Take sips of hot water
- Get up slowly in the morning and, if at all possible, rest during the day
- Avoid any smells which you know make you want to vomit
- Wear travel sickness bands
- Ask an acupuncturist to show you the pressure point on your hand which controls sickness.

ACHES AND PAINS IN PREGNANCY

Piles (Haemorrhoids)

Piles are varicose veins in your back passage and can make opening your bowels very painful. Lots of women find it too embarrassing to ask for help with this problem, which is quite understandable, although your doctor or midwife will be used to advising women about haemorrhoids. You can try the following:

- Have a high fibre diet rich in wholemeal bread, jacket potatoes, fruit and vegetables
- Don't put off going to the toilet to open your bowels; if you feel the urge to go, go!
- Drink lots of water
- Practise your pelvic floor exercises regularly
- Take plenty of exercise generally
- Go to a reputable shop selling herbal remedies and ask for herbal pile tablets.

Stretch Marks

There's no scientific evidence that any of the creams which you can buy over the counter will help you avoid getting stretch marks if that is the way your body responds to pregnancy, but some women find that rubbing cream into their breasts, stomach and thighs makes them feel more comfortable.

If these same women avoid stretch marks no one can say whether it was the cream or their bodies that did the trick! The cream will certainly soothe the dry skin that pregnancy can cause. Be assured that after your baby is born, the red lines will become silvery and much less noticeable.

- Ask an aromatherapist to prescribe you an oil to reduce the vividness of the stretch lines after your baby is born
- Vitamin E cream may also help postnatally.

special attention which they receive. Pregnancy says very important things about you. It announces that you are really 'grown-up', have obviously been sexually active, are capable of conceiving a child, will soon be facing labour, and in a few months, will be taking responsibility for the 24–hour-a-day care of a new baby:

'When I was pregnant I felt really special, really proud, walking around with my bump. If ever we went out, to the pictures or the pub, I'd be sticking my tummy out; I wanted everybody to know. When I was three months pregnant, we went to France on a camping holiday and I was telling everyone I was pregnant. It wasn't that noticeable, of course, but I just wanted everybody to know. I felt so confident. Being pregnant gives a real boost to your confidence.'

'I was not totally happy about the weight I was putting on, but I did feel very proud of myself. Pregnancy gave me a new sense of self-respect.'

PELVIC FLOOR EXERCISES

These are really important! At the bottom of your pelvis is a big sling of muscles which keep your bladder, womb and back passage in their right places and help them to function well. During pregnancy, these muscles become very stretched because of the increased weight which they are supporting and because of pregnancy hormones which make them slack. As a result, you may find that you start to wet yourself a little when you cough or sneeze or laugh. Like any other muscles in your body, your pelvic floor muscles need exercising if they are to remain strong. Some women find that, because their pelvic floor muscles are weak, they suffer a prolapse in their middle years. You can help yourself avoid problems now and in later life if you learn and then practise daily some simple exercises.

- Put your clenched fist to your mouth and cough into it. You should be able to feel your pelvic floor muscles bulging between your legs. These are the muscles you're going to exercise
- Tighten the muscles around your back passage and then the muscles at the front around your vagina as if you're trying to stop yourself from passing wind. Then tighten them more and more, imagining that you have a lift between your legs and you are taking it up to the first floor and then the second and then the third. When you are at the third floor, your muscles should be as tight as if you desperately need to go to the toilet but have to hold on for a while
- Try to continue to breathe while you are tightening the muscles!
- Now, in stages, relax the muscles so that you come down to the second floor and then the first and then the ground floor. Don't let them crash from the third floor down to the ground!
- Try making the muscles bulge now by pushing them down to the basement. You will need to be able to do this when you are pushing your baby out into the world in the second part of labour
- Finish the exercise by returning the muscles to their normal state on the ground floor.

Repeat this exercise a few times, tightening the muscles in stages, breathing all the time, and then letting the muscles relax in stages.

In order to exercise all the different fibres which make up your pelvic floor muscles, you also need to do the following exercise:

- Draw your muscles up as tight as you can between your legs and hold for one second; then relax them. Repeat this 10 times.

Pelvic floor muscles need to be exercised daily. To help yourself remember, do them each time you: have a drink, wash something up, brush your hair, stop at red traffic lights, look in a mirror, or every time you do anything which you have to do several times a day!

The best way of testing your pelvic floor muscles is during love-making. Your partner will be able to tell you how strong they are!

It's not a good idea to test your muscles by trying to stop the flow of urine when you are on the toilet. Although women used to be told to do this, it's now thought to cause problems because some women can't get going again after stopping the flow. However, it is a good idea to do your pelvic floor muscle exercises *after* you've used the toilet when your bladder is empty. If you are doing the exercises each time you go to the loo, you should be practising them sufficiently.

EATING AND DRINKING IN PREGNANCY

There has been so much publicity about what women should and should not eat during pregnancy that you may feel very nervous about how best to look after yourself and your baby in this respect. Whilst it is not a good idea to eat for two, pregnancy can be a time when you make a special effort to enjoy a healthy, varied diet with plenty of basic foods such as bread, potatoes, cereals, fruit and vegetables. In fact, there are only a few things which you need to avoid:

● Soft cheeses such as Brie and Camembert
● Blue-veined cheeses such as Stilton and Danish Blue
● Raw and soft boiled eggs
● Pate and liver sausage
● Undercooked meat and poultry which is still pink
● Unwrapped foods such as sausage rolls which you are not going to heat through thoroughly
● Ready-to-eat poultry
● Coleslaw and pre-prepared salads.

The chances of catching listeria or salmonella from these foods are probably very small, but there is a slight risk and you can still eat well without having to take any risk at all.

● Liver. If you eat a lot of liver, there is a danger that you will overdose on vitamin A which could be harmful to your baby. However, eating liver once or twice during your pregnancy is not going to do any harm.

If you feel concerned about what you have eaten or drunk, talk to your midwife or ring the Eating for Pregnancy Helpline on 01142 424084.

The debate about how much alcohol it is safe for pregnant women to drink is still raging. While some women who drink moderately, and more who drink a lot, run the risk of having a baby who is damaged by alcohol, the risk for those who drink only a few glasses of wine or spirits a week is hard to calculate. Some people feel that having a drink in the evening helps them to relax and a relaxed mother is probably better able to help her baby grow well in the uterus (womb) than one who is very tense. The following guidelines, therefore, seem to be generally accepted:

● If you are at the stage of planning a baby, cut out alcohol until you are twelve weeks pregnant

● Avoid drinking heavily in early pregnancy. If you did go on a 'binge' before you knew you were pregnant, don't have another, but try not to worry too much as the research about binge drinking doesn't prove that it's harmful to babies (although it does suggest that it's not a good idea)

● If you enjoy a drink, stick to one drink a day. A single glass of wine, half a pint of lager or a small whisky, for example, is almost certainly not going to cause your baby any problems and may be important in helping you relax and enjoy your pregnancy.

EXERCISE IN PREGNANCY

If you enjoyed exercising before you became pregnant, there is no reason why you should not continue to do so as long as both you and your baby are healthy. One sport which is definitely not a good idea for a pregnant woman is deep-sea diving. If diving is your sport, you should not dive below 18 metres during your pregnancy.

There are a few precautions to bear in mind:

- Pregnancy is not the time to take up vigorous exercise which you have not been used to before

- If your body tells you that you are overdoing it, or you start to have aches and pains while exercising, give yourself a break

- Have plenty to drink before you start exercising and avoid taking exercise in hot weather. Pregnant women get dehydrated very easily (which is why you should avoid saunas in pregnancy)

- Competitive sportswomen who want to train right up to the time their baby is born, should check with their doctor that this is all right. Some researchers have found that women who are exercising at a very high level during the last weeks of their pregnancy give birth to babies with low birthweights.

In general, a woman who is fit because exercising is a regular part of her life is likely to be well prepared to cope with the demands of labour.

Your partner's attitude to you may well change; he may register his anxiety about your well-being and the well-being of his baby by increased caution and concern: *'It's a special time and my husband treated me differently – very caringly. Not that he isn't normally caring; he was just even more so.'*

Even though they are not carrying the baby themselves, partners have to live with someone who is. Men are often surprised to find how emotional the woman is during her pregnancy:

'I've found it hard to cope with her general irritability, forgetfulness and paranoia.'

'She's so worried about birth pain that she's got me really worried too.'

The change in their partner's shape can also cause anxiety:

'I'm worried all the time about not bumping into her.'

'She is enormous, *simply enormous! Is that normal?'*

For women, labour is a hurdle it is difficult to see beyond, but men tend to think ahead to the time after the birth, and wonder how things will change when the couple becomes a family: *'I don't know how we'll handle the changes in our lives. Our relationship will change. We'll have less money.'*

INFECTIONS IN PREGNANCY

Many women find that, once the first three months of their pregnancy are over, they feel exceptionally well and remain so until the birth of their babies. Coughs and colds are always around, and you don't need to worry if you catch a cold, although you have every excuse to pamper yourself if you do feel unwell! There are a few infections which can cause problems:

Rubella (German Measles): if a woman catches rubella at the beginning of her pregnancy there is a strong likelihood that her baby will be born with serious problems affecting his sight and hearing. The later in pregnancy the virus is caught, the less dangerous it is for the baby. Your rubella immunity should be routinely checked at the beginning of your pregnancy and you should ask your doctor or midwife to tell you the result.

Varicella Zoster (Chickenpox): when a woman catches chickenpox in the first half of pregnancy, her baby may be born with scars from the infection and is sometimes mentally disabled. The baby is also at risk if the mother catches chickenpox just before she is due to give birth. A mother who has chickenpox needs to see her doctor because there are treatments available which may help reduce the effect of the virus on her baby.

Toxoplasmosis: toxoplasmosis in this country is most commonly caught from handling cat litter or eating undercooked meat. If the mother becomes infected during the first half of her pregnancy, her baby may be born too early or may have a disability.

You can help protect yourself from toxoplasmosis in these ways:

● Always cook meat thoroughly
● Wash your hands after handling raw meat, and wash down any work surfaces which the raw meat has touched
● Wear gloves for gardening and wash home-grown vegetables or bought vegetables before eating them
● Wear rubber gloves to empty cat litter trays.

Human Immunodeficiency Virus (HIV): women who are HIV positive run a high risk of transmitting the virus to their babies, and should receive special counselling to help them consider their choices in pregnancy, for birth and after their babies are born.

Those who are uncertain about their new role as father and perhaps unsure about whether they really want a baby may protect themselves from anxiety during the pregnancy by refusing to anticipate what the future holds: *'I think Roy's pleased but very wary; he won't think about the baby until it comes.'*

Unfortunately, a father generally has far fewer opportunities to talk through his feelings about pregnancy than his partner. Encouragement and support for men who are expecting a baby, facing labour or going through early parenthood are sadly lacking in our society.

Feeling different and different feelings

THE FIRST THREE months of pregnancy are often extremely tiring. The baby is growing at an almost unimaginable rate even though there is no bump to show yet. His world is microscopic, but deep inside your pelvis, cells are dividing and multiplying and being set aside in groups to become brain, heart, liver, digestive tract, kidneys, arms, legs and face in a manner that is positively frantic. It is no wonder that many women feel exhausted at the beginning of pregnancy.

Morning sickness is common during these first months; some women simply *feel* sick – not just in the morning, but at all times of the day and night – and some spend a lot of time being sick. Other people may not take it very seriously: after all, morning sickness is just the price you have to pay for being pregnant. It means more than that to some women, however, who find that they can no longer eat the foods they once enjoyed and crave for things that they would never have eaten before they were pregnant. Such major changes in eating habits really bring home to you that something very dramatic is happening to your body: *'Prior to getting pregnant, I had just started to try and slim down and get fit. The healthy eating stopped when the nausea began. The thought of salads and anything green remained repulsive to me throughout my pregnancy. I felt sick for twenty weeks, although it was more bearable after fifteen.'*

The physical changes which pregnancy brings about make some women feel very out of control of themselves and they have to adjust to being not quite their own person any more: *'Watching my body change without me influencing it, being examined by doctors and midwives on a regular basis, meant having to cope with a new sense of myself.'*

MISCARRIAGE

HEALTH PROFESSIONALS call the loss of a baby before 24 weeks of pregnancy a miscarriage and after this time, a stillbirth. For the woman involved, how long she has been pregnant makes very little difference: *'I was thirteen weeks. They said it was an early miscarriage – it didn't feel like an early miscarriage to me.'*

A miscarriage often starts with bleeding from the vagina and period-like pains, but it may be days or weeks before the woman is certain that she is going to lose her baby: *'When the bleeding started, I felt I knew the end result, but waiting a week to find out on the scan definitely seemed an eternity. The scan showed the baby had died at eleven weeks. There was nothing anybody could do to lessen the blow.'*

'I'd had three weeks of fluid loss and uncertainty and I finally went in at 17 weeks with a prolapsed cord and that was it. I had the children with me so we decided to take them to mum's and go back to hospital and they induced me that night. Having had three weeks of ups and downs – was it OK, wasn't it? – I guess I just wanted it to be finished.'

Although a miscarriage which happens before 12 weeks may feel only like a particularly uncomfortable period, if the miscarriage happens later, the woman may have to go into hospital to give birth to her dead baby. Being in hospital may well be very distressing: *'It's very depressing having women on the ward with you who are pregnant and just having bed rest and I cried my eyes out when I heard them listening to the baby's heartbeat in the next bed, knowing that I wasn't going to have a baby.'*

Some women choose to go home first, and to spend a few days preparing themselves before they come into hospital for the labour: *'When we went for my scan, he was dead and we didn't know. I mean he*

MISCARRIAGE

(losing a baby before 24 weeks of pregnancy)

What to look for:

Bleeding from the vagina – brownish spots or bright red bleeding
Pain – period-like pains which come and go
Backache – low down in the back

What to do:

- Contact your midwife or doctor and ask for advice
- Rest or continue with light activities, whichever you would rather do (there is no proof that lying in bed helps prevent a miscarriage, although this is often recommended and may make you feel better)
- Don't have intercourse while the bleeding continues
- Ask your partner, a good friend, or your mum, to come and be with you.

What will happen:

- You have to wait and see – which is the hardest part of all
- If the bleeding continues and gets heavier, a miscarriage is probably inevitable
- If you have a lot of severe pain and very heavy bleeding, you may be taken into hospital to be cared for until the miscarriage happens
- The bleeding may get less and the pregnancy continue quite normally.

Looking after *you*

Whatever happens, whether you lose the baby or the pregnancy settles down again, you will have had a great shock and need and deserve lots of support:

- Find a friend you can talk to about what's happened (your partner may be as shocked as you and not able to support you at this time)
- Ask your midwife or doctor to explain anything you don't understand
- Contact the Miscarriage Association or The National Childbirth Trust and ask to be put in touch with someone who can support you.

kicked that morning and I went for my 20 week scan and he was dead. They said, "We can induce labour now or you can go home and prepare yourself and we suggest you go home." And that was what I wanted – time to think about what had happened and what would happen.'

Telling other people about the miscarriage adds an extra dimension to the trauma, especially if children need to be told: *'Telling our daughter was very difficult as she had been so looking forward to the new baby.'*

However, children generally accept events more readily than adults who often find it very hard to know how to respond to such distressing news: *'Perhaps they were frightened of upsetting me, but when they made no comment about the miscarriage, or later when I met them in the street, they just gave me a sidewards glance, I felt as if I had done something wrong and it was all my fault.'*

What parents who have miscarried their baby need more than anything is to have their loss acknowledged: *'A few words would have been far better than none.'*

THE SECOND HALF OF PREGNANCY

IN THE SECOND half of pregnancy, as the bump starts to get bigger, problems which are related to the woman's increasing weight such as aching legs and cramps, varicose veins and piles may occur. The hormones of pregnancy make the valve at the top of the stomach less efficient and acid from the stomach may wash back into the gullet and cause heartburn. Most women, if they have people to support them, are able to cope well with these discomforts, but they can nonetheless be very unpleasant: *'The constipation that had been an ongoing feature of my pregnancy got worse and I started to suffer quite badly with piles. The fibre boosters from the GP just about got me going, but because I had gone off vegetables as soon as I became pregnant and because drinking fruit juice gave me heartburn, there wasn't much I could do to help myself and I just had to grin and bear it.'*

Women are keen to look after themselves while they are pregnant and it is a time when many reassess their lives and try to become more health conscious. Something which might have been much too difficult to do when you were not pregnant, such as giving up smoking or taking regular exercise, suddenly becomes possible when you know that your baby will benefit from the healthier lifestyle. New eating habits, having more rest, and making an effort to swim or walk a couple of times a week bring with them a feeling of well-being.

'I felt healthier by the day. I ate decent food and read and relaxed.'

'The swimming made me very fit and I had no problems carrying my ever growing bump.'

The middle part of a first pregnancy may be one of the most enjoyable times of a woman's life. The labour is still sufficiently far in the future not to cause too much concern. There is the excitement of first feeling the baby moving and later on, the undeniable reality of the baby kicking vigorously at all times of the day and night!

'I loved my growing belly and spent hours stroking it and wondering what the baby would be like.'

Towards the end of pregnancy, the tiredness which was a feature of the first few weeks reappears. Being pregnant and still having to go to

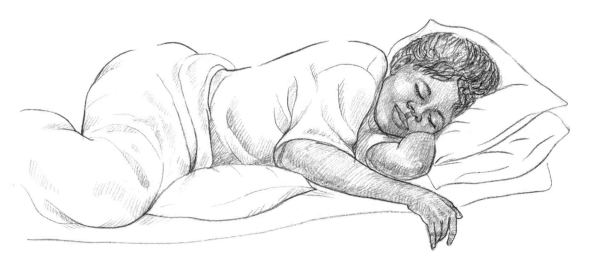

YOUR BABY'S GROWTH AND DEVELOPMENT

First Three Months of Pregnancy

- Your baby grows very quickly
- His heart begins to beat
- His blood is circulating round his body
- He can suck, swallow and wee
- His arms and legs start to form
- His face begins to develop its unique appearance
- He starts to move.

Second Three Months of Pregnancy

- Now you start to feel your baby first stirring and then moving more vigorously inside you
- Your baby's heart can be heard by the midwife with an ear trumpet through the wall of your tummy (or by you if you ask to use a stethoscope)
- The two sections which form the hard palate inside your baby's mouth join together

- Your baby's fingernails start to grow
- He is developing his own pattern of sleeping and waking and you are learning to recognise when he is active and when he is resting
- He can hear and will 'jump' if there is a sudden loud noise
- His eyes are open.

The Last Three Months of Pregnancy

- Your baby now starts to make breathing movements
- His skin becomes smoother and less wrinkled and hairy
- His nails and hair grow longer and his skull hardens
- His body becomes rounder and plumper as he lays down fat ready for labour and the first few days of his life.

---

work are an exhausting combination and many women long for the day when their maternity leave will begin: *'I could no longer cope with the journey to work by train – three changes, so I used to leave home in the car at 7am to miss the traffic, go swimming at the leisure centre near the office, and get to work in time to eat breakfast.'*

It is during the last three months of pregnancy that some women find themselves monopolising all the pillows in the house at night to put one under the bump, one between their legs, one in the small of their back and a couple under their head in an effort to be sufficiently comfortable to get to sleep. Turning over in bed becomes a major undertaking, and partners may decide that they stand a better chance of getting some continuous rest if they retire to the sofa or the spare room for a while!

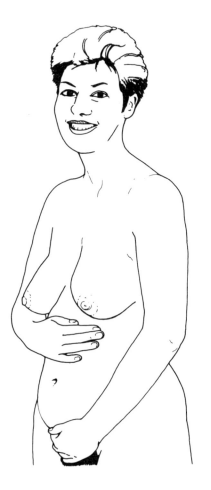

THE NINE MONTHS MIRACLE – THE FIRST TRIMESTER

Although your baby may seem to grow up very quickly after he is born, never again will he grow and change as quickly as he did in your womb. When you have been pregnant for three weeks, your baby is about the size of a pea, just a cluster of cells which contain within them the amazing potential to become a fully formed human individual who will be uniquely your child. By the time you are 12 weeks pregnant – with no bump yet to show! – your baby is the size of an avocado pear but his heart and blood vessels, kidneys, gut, sexual organs, nervous system, head and face, arms and legs are all formed. His heart is beating, his blood is flowing round his body and he can suck, swallow and wee.

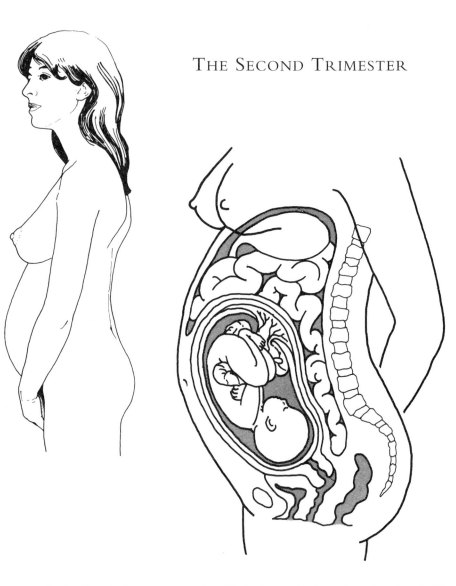

THE SECOND TRIMESTER

During the rest of your pregnancy, he will simply grow in size and practise using the different parts of his body. You will be able to feel him moving from when you are about 18–22 weeks pregnant if this is your first pregnancy, or earlier if this is your second pregnancy but your baby has really been moving since he was two months old. By five months of pregnancy, your baby can hear your voice – talk to him; try to remember the nursery rhymes you once knew! By six and a half months, his eyes are open and as your tummy stretches, he can distinguish light from dark.

The Third Trimester

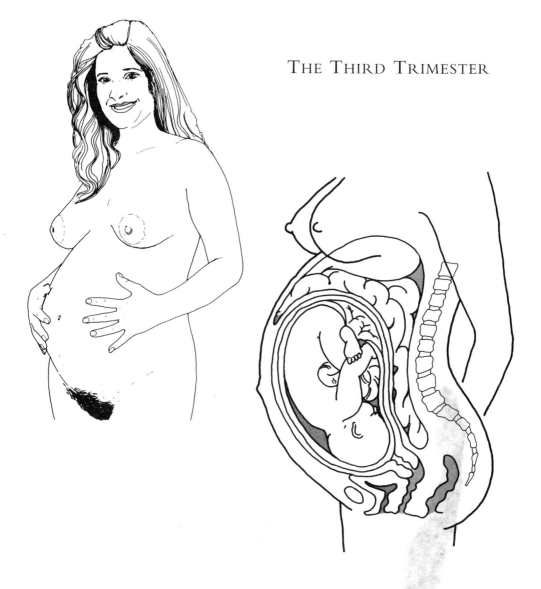

During his last three months in the womb, your baby's nails will grow to reach the end of his fingertips – and beyond – and his hair gets longer. He becomes much fatter as he prepares for the hard work of being born and adjusting to life in the outside world.

DRUGS IN PREGNANCY

Street Drugs

Much of the research about what happens to babies when their mothers use street drugs during pregnancy has included only small numbers of women and their babies. There is also a lack of research to differentiate between women who regularly use street drugs and those who are occasional users. So our understanding of street drugs and pregnancy is limited in some important ways. That said, there seems to be little doubt that street drugs cause all sorts of problems for babies. Nobody is likely to have an unborn baby's interests more at heart than the woman who is carrying him. If a pregnant woman is using an illegal drug, the best thing she can do for her baby is to get some help. At the end of this book are addresses of agencies which offer confidential and non-judgemental counselling and advice.

What follows is a list of some of the risks which babies run if their mothers are taking illegal drugs.

Amphetamines and Ecstasy
Babies are at risk of:
● Being born too early
● Being born very small
● Having a cleft palate
● Having heart problems
● Having a mental disability.

Cannabis
Babies are at risk of:
● Being born too early
● Being very hppy and difficult to settle in the first : of their lives
● Develop wly in the first years of life.

At the mom research into cannabis has not linked i h higher rates of disability amongst ba born to mothers who smoke regularly.

Cocaine
Babies are at :
● Dying in the cause their mothers develop ser d pressure problems
● Being born w. renous toes and fingers
● Having heart ar. problems
● Being extremely i e in the first weeks of life and requiring s cial nursing to help them cope with withd al symptoms.

It is absolutely certain that even women who are not addicted to cocaine and use it only occasionally are putting their babies at serious risk.

Heroin
Babies are at risk of:
● Being born too early
● Being very small and sickly
● Needing treatment to help them cope with withdrawal symptoms
● Developing slowly both physically and mentally in the first years of life.

LSD
It's still not certain what effect LSD has on unborn and newborn babies. There doesn't seem to be a higher rate of abnormality amongst babies born to women who use LSD. However, the substances which often contaminate illegal LSD may be dangerous for babies.

Solvents and Glue
Babies are at risk of:
● Being very small and short at birth
● Having kidney and bladder problems.

Methadone
Methadone is legally available in this country to heroin addicts and addicts of other drugs. It carries its own risks. Women who use methadone are more likely to miscarry and their babies, if they survive, are slow to develop in the first years of life. However, they do appear to catch up with other 'normal' children by the time they are two or three years old.

DRUGS IN PREGNANCY

Over the Counter Drugs

Most people take drugs on a daily basis – aspirin and paracetamol, cough mixtures and cold remedies, laxatives and caffeine – and never think that they are using drugs. A quick look in the medicine cupboard at home will probably show lots of tablets and mixtures bought from the pharmacy at some time, many of them now out of date. You may have bottles with no labels on them and you can't quite remember what they contain. Pregnancy is a good time to go through your medicine cabinet and throw away anything you are uncertain about.

While there are, in fact, very few over the counter or prescription drugs which are defi-

nitely known to be harmful to unborn babies (and some of these are drugs which women have to continue to take when they are pregnant such as drugs for epilepsy), it is wise to be cautious during pregnancy. Ask your doctor or local pharmacist (pharmacists are often undervalued as a source of excellent, up-to-date information on drugs) about any tablet or medicine you are thinking of taking. Cut down on drinks containing caffeine (mainly coffee and cola). Continue to be careful until your baby is born or, if you are breastfeeding, until your baby is not feeding from you any longer. Whatever drugs you are taking, your unborn or breast-feeding baby will have to take them as well.

WAITING FOR LABOUR TO START

PREGNANCY AND ESPECIALLY late pregnancy are full of dreams and imaginings about what the baby will be like. For most people, there is considerable anxiety about whether the baby will be healthy. Fears of having a baby who is not normal or who is born dead can cause a lot of distress: *'I have a recurring nightmare that I'm giving birth and the baby gets stuck inside me and the midwife yanks him out and he's dead.'*

'I'm going to accept whatever comes along in labour as long as the baby and I are OK. Of course, I have an ideal birth in my mind and an ideal baby – hopefully they will happen.'

Some women daren't allow themselves to think too much about labour in case the

SMOKING IN PREGNANCY

Sadly, mothers who smoke during pregnancy and after their babies are born are not doing either themselves or their babies any good. Smoking reduces the supply of oxygen to the baby while he is in the uterus. Babies are more likely to die in the womb or at birth if their mothers smoke; they can be born prematurely and are sometimes small and sickly. After birth, these babies are at greater risk of cot death because they are living in a smoky environment.

Sometimes it's too hard for women to give up smoking even though they are anxious to do what is right for their babies. So:

● If you can give up, do
● If you think you could give up, get all the help you can from your GP, from your midwife, from your partner and friends
● If you simply can't give up, try to cut down; every cigarette you don't smoke is going to be good for your baby.

baby is not born healthy: *'I don't think about the birth in case something goes wrong; it's like a barrier, a defence I have put up.'*

Others, however, seem to be always serene and confident: *'I have never for a moment wondered whether the baby will be OK. I just know he will. I often put headphones on my stomach and play the baby music and talk about the things we'll do together.'*

It can be difficult to imagine what you will feel like when your baby is born and first put into your arms. During pregnancy, the baby has a fantasy life which means that she can be whatever her mother wants her to be; as the moment of birth approaches, women have to come to terms with replacing the fantasy with reality:

'I try not to think about how I'll feel when I meet my baby; I might be disappointed, so I'll just wait and see what happens at the time with no big expectations. It could be one extreme or the other.'

'I really love my baby already. Whether I'll feel like that when it's born, I'm not sure.'

Some people would strongly prefer to have a baby of one sex or the other and the end of pregnancy is the time when it becomes necessary to accept the fact that such a dream may not be realised: *'Every time I've dreamt about the baby, it's been a boy. I think it's something to do with the fact that we'd both like a girl, so I think it's my way of trying to come to terms with the fact that it might be a boy.'*

ONCE LABOUR is only a few weeks away, women start to face up to the business of giving birth. It is likely that they will have heard a lot of stories about labour – and perhaps been very frightened by some of them. Women can be unconsciously unkind to other women who have not yet had babies when they describe and perhaps exaggerate the trials of their labours. Nonetheless, it is probably true that women at all times and in all cultures have looked forward to labour with a mixture of eager anticipation and dread:

'You don't know what you are going to feel.'

'I'm trying to be positive about it all; I don't really know what it is going to feel like. I think it might be like going for a long walk up a mountain when you don't know if you're getting near to the top.'

'I'm not looking forward to the labour and birth. I'm worried about how painful it's going to be. I'm looking forward to after the birth when I've got the baby.'

'It can't be that bad or the population of the planet would have stopped.'

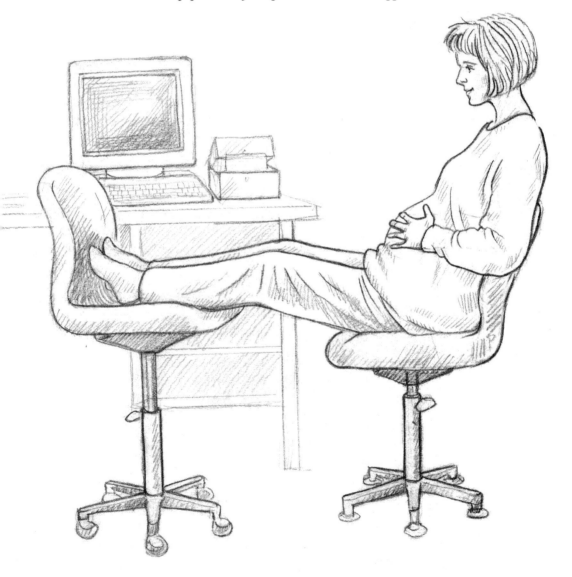

When the day on which the baby is due to be born arrives and passes without anything happening, women find themselves the objects of sometimes unwanted attention as friends and relatives start ringing to ask whether the baby has come yet. The last few weeks can seem very long and many women become anxious for labour to start: *'It somehow seems better if it comes early. Waiting for labour, especially when it's late, feels dreadful. You feel so big and uncomfortable, you can't sleep. There's the excitement as well – thinking you might be having contractions; then they go away and you realise that it wasn't* IT *!'*

'I really enjoyed the last few weeks of my pregnancy pottering about. My due date came and so did my mother who was going to look after us after the birth, but the baby didn't. Every day, Michael and mum would empty and refill the

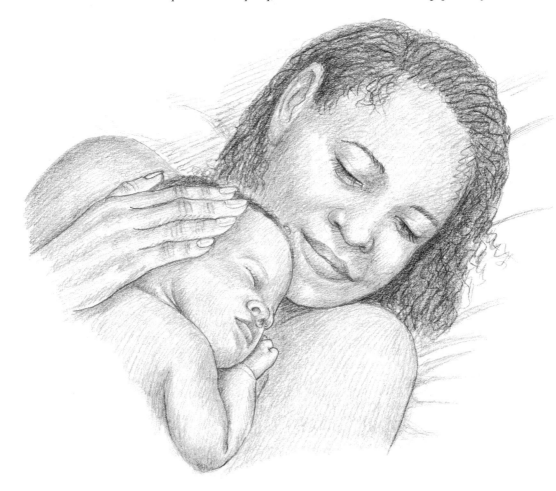

*birthing pool and get everything ready to go. I felt as if I was in limbo. I
didn't really believe that I was actually going to meet the baby inside me.'*

MANY WOMEN – and more men! – are frightened that they will not
recognise when labour has started. Talking to other parents and to
midwives and health professionals, reading books and going to antenatal classes help to give you an idea of what to expect. Although you
may have false alarms and think you are in labour when you are not,
eventually the day will come when you are quite sure: *'I remember
everyone saying that I would know when labour had started and not believing
them. But I did!'*

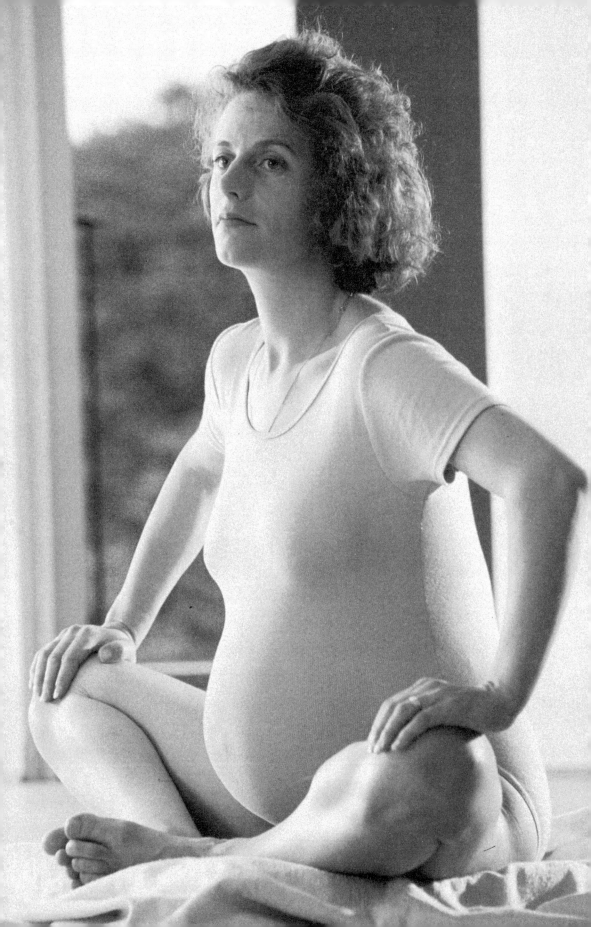

CHAPTER *two* *Choosing where your baby will be born*

HOW DO PEOPLE make choices about health care? How, for example, does a pregnant woman decide whether her baby should be born at home or in hospital? There are all sorts of influences at work upon her, some of which she will be aware of and some of which will affect her quite unconsciously. She may be influenced by what she has seen on television and at the cinema and by newspaper articles, magazines and books she has read. Perhaps more significantly, she might be influenced by her own mother and where she had her babies. If her mother had home births and enjoyed them, or had hospital births and felt very satisfied there, she might feel that she will be happy with the same thing:

'I think because my mother had all of us at home, a home birth seemed a natural choice for me.'

'I was born in hospital, even though it was less common then than it is now, and my mother had no problems at all.'

A woman may be influenced by the experiences which her sister(s) or other relatives have had. The stories she is told by her close friends about the local hospitals or about home births may have a profound influence on her: *'My friend had a Domino delivery and had a very positive experience and I'm sure that influenced me.'*

'My sisters had their babies in hospital and it just seemed that they had one intervention after another and that put me off having my baby in hospital. I didn't want to get on a conveyor belt.'

'I went to the local hospital because my two closest girlfriends had their babies there in the last couple of years and it was just a lovely hospital.'

MOST WOMEN choose to give birth in hospital because they think hospital is the safest place for a baby to be born. The same view does not necessarily hold amongst women in other countries; in Holland, for example, it has been and still is quite usual to give birth at home and the government provides women with home nurses for a few weeks after they have delivered their babies. By contrast, government policy in the UK from 1970 to the early 1990s was to aim for 100% hospital delivery. In 1993, however, an Expert Maternity Group set up by the government, concluded that there is no clear statistical evidence that having babies away from general hospital maternity units is any less safe for women with uncomplicated pregnancies. It may be that society will now reconsider its attitude towards home birth, and that more women will choose this option as doctors and midwives start explaining to them that it is fine to have their babies at home.

GETTING INFORMATION AND BECOMING CONFIDENT

IF WOMEN want to make choices about the kind of care they receive in pregnancy and during labour, they may have to do some, if not all, of the work of finding out what's available for themselves. In the beginning, you may not know exactly what you want when you go to your GP to discuss your pregnancy and the birth of your baby. You may have no idea about the different kinds of care available to you; you may never have had anything to do with hospitals in your life, never have had any medical tests, never have spoken to a midwife, never have held a newborn baby. However, you will soon become very much more aware simply because once you are pregnant, you start to take note of items on the television and in the newspapers about birth and babies and you start to have conversations with friends who have had babies; you go to clinics where you talk to other pregnant women about the decisions they have made and attend antenatal classes where there is heaps of information on offer:

'This is my first pregnancy and there's such a lot I don't know about. Going to the classes and talking through all the choices and options with other women and the teacher have been a very important part of thinking about the sort of birth I want.'

YOUR CHOICES FOR MATERNITY CARE

Ask yourself:

- Would you prefer to receive most of your ante and postnatal care at your GP's surgery, and go to the hospital just once or twice during your pregnancy, and then to give birth to your baby in the Consultant Unit? (This is called 'shared care'.)

  If you have a GP Unit at your local maternity hospital, your GP may be able to care for you there when your baby is born or you can be looked after by the hospital midwives.

  Some GPs are willing to book you for a home birth and to provide all your maternity care before, during and after the birth of your baby. (However, you don't have to have a GP cover you for a home birth. A midwife has the legal right and practical skills to take sole responsibility for your maternity care provided no complications arise.)

- Would you prefer to receive most of your ante and postnatal care from a small team of midwives whom you can get to know and one of whom will help you give birth? (Most areas are now starting to organise midwives into teams so this should be a real option for you.)

- Would you prefer to receive care from a community midwife who will look after you during your pregnancy, go into hospital with you to help you give birth and then accompany you home with your baby a few hours afterwards?

  This is called the Domino scheme. It's not available everywhere; you need to ask your midwife or the Director of Maternity Services at your local Maternity Unit about having this kind of care.

  There are increasing numbers of hospital-based schemes running now which arrange for each mother to be cared for by just one midwife. Ask if such a scheme is running at your hospital.

- Would you prefer to receive most of your care from the obstetricians at the local maternity hospital and attend antenatal clinics there whilst receiving postnatal care from the community midwives?

- Would you like to employ an independent midwife to care for you throughout your pregnancy and labour until a few weeks after your baby is born?

Suddenly you will be inundated with information and very able to decide for yourself about such things as where to have your baby. If, in the middle or even at the end of your pregnancy, you want to change your mind about decisions that were taken at the start of your pregnancy, there is no reason why you should not: *'When we went to book at the Health Centre, the doctor said to me: "You're over thirty so you won't want to have your baby at home. Your options are to go to hospital a, b or c." I said, "Oh yes, that's fine." Later on, I became quite worried because*

I don't like hospitals and someone mentioned home birth so I started finding out about it. I went to a home birth support group meeting; suddenly everything felt right and I decided to go for it.'

MAKING CHOICES IN DIFFICULT CIRCUMSTANCES

IT'S LARGELY a question of confidence when it comes to making decisions – confidence that you know what is right for you: *'To get the choices you want, you don't ask, you just say. But you have to feel confident.'*

Feeling confident is very hard, however, if you've had previous experience of a birth that was difficult. In these circumstances, women often choose to have a different type of care from what they might once have preferred: *'I wanted a home birth with my first pregnancy and was amazed at the opposition I had. But then I had a late miscarriage and moved to a different area and home wasn't really home. I felt panic-stricken when I became pregnant again. All my priorities changed completely and I thought, "I don't care where this baby is born as long as it's born alive." When I met the GP for the first time, she assumed that I'd want all the technology available and home birth wasn't discussed. It was just a case of booking me in to the hospital and keeping a really close eye on me. I was really pleased with that.'*

'I had a mass of interventions during my first labour; one just led to another and then another. I'm very anxious to avoid all of that this time. I'd quite like a home birth and not to go near a hospital, but, on the other hand, because I needed all those interventions first time round, there's a part of me that wouldn't like to risk a home birth. So I've chosen a Domino delivery.'

In cases such as these, decisions depend on weighing up what you would ideally like against what will make you feel most secure. As long as the final choice is yours, you are likely to feel more satisfied with it than if someone else had made it for you.

Choosing a home birth

WOMEN WHO choose to have a home birth give all sorts of reasons for their decision. Some simply know in their heart of hearts that this is

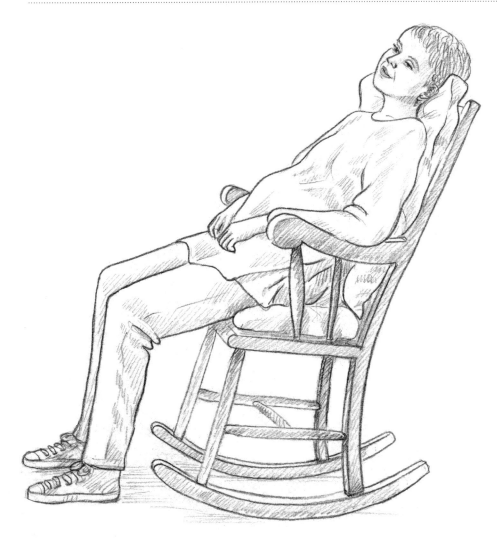

where their baby should be born; others feel that they will be more relaxed in their own home; some cherish the privacy which they can have at home and the freedom to do as they choose; some find hospitals frightening and fear that they are likely to have a lot of inter- ventions if they have their babies there:

'I've chosen a home birth. I want as few interventions as possible. I'd like assistance – a LOT of assistance but as few interventions as possible.'

'One of the main reasons I wanted to have my baby at home is that I felt if I went into hospital with strangers around, I wouldn't be very assertive. I

WHERE DO YOU WANT YOUR BABY TO BE BORN?

This is an important decision which you will be asked to make at the beginning of your pregnancy – although you can change your mind later on if you want to. Key questions to consider are:

Home Birth

- Will you be more relaxed in labour if you are in your own home where you can do what you please?
- Would you prefer the midwife to be a guest in your house rather than being the midwife's 'guest' at the hospital?
- Will you feel safer at home?
- Do you want to have as little medical intervention during your labour as possible?
- How does your partner feel about home birth?
- Is your home suitable for you to give birth there? (Is there a telephone? Is there somewhere you can be quiet? Is there heating in the room where the baby will be born? Is there a private toilet and hot water? Can you make arrangements for your other children to be cared for elsewhere if you don't want them to be present at the birth?)

Hospital Birth

- Will you be more relaxed in labour if you are in hospital where there are doctors and midwives always around?
- Will you feel safer in hospital?
- How does your partner feel about hospital birth?
- Will the hospital help you to have the kind of birth you want to have?

If you choose to have your baby in hospital, you might want to consider which hospital to book at if there are several in your area. Ask yourself:

- What have you heard about the local maternity units from other women who have recently given birth? This kind of information is invaluable – women who have given birth at a particular hospital *really* know what it is like!
- Does one hospital or one consultant have a reputation for using a lot of medical procedures during labour and another a reputation for letting women do what they want?

  Which attitude would suit you better? You should be able to get statistics about such things as how many women have their labours induced, and how many women have forceps delivery or caesarean sections at each of your local maternity units from:

  (i)   the hospitals themselves
  (ii) your local Maternity Services Liaison Committee
  (iii) the Community Health Council

  You can also enquire about the intervention rates of individual consultant obstetricians.
  You might want to take this kind of information into account when choosing between hospitals and consultants.

- How easy is it for you to get to each of the local hospitals?
- Is there one which seems better maintained, more up to date and more comfortable?
- Are some units keen to send women home quickly after their babies are born simply because there are too few beds on the postnatal wards?
- Do any of the local units have a birthing pool so that you can use water to help you cope with pain in labour?

thought that if the midwife was coming into my house, she'd be far more likely to ask me before doing something.'

'The thing about home birth is having a one-to-one relationship with the midwife. The midwife who walks through my door will be with me throughout the whole of my labour.'

'I can have candlelight if I want to. I can wander around the house making as much noise as I like! Everything I need is here.'

'I knew instinctively that I wanted my babies at home.'

'I wasn't really sure why I wanted to have my baby at home, but I could see no reason to go into hospital and I used to get annoyed when people asked, "Why are you having it at home?" I'd just say, "Why not?"'

If your partner is going to support you during labour, or you have asked someone else to be with you, it is essential that they are happy with your choice of a home birth. Someone who is frightened of the environment in which you have decided to labour, either because it's too clinical or because it's not clinical enough, will almost certainly not be able to give you the reassurance and support which you need. Talking through where you want your baby to be born and allowing your chosen labour supporter to gather his own information will often result in a mutually acceptable decision: *'My partner wasn't so keen on the home birth idea. I explained to him my thinking and let him talk to other people about home births. I didn't push him. I didn't want him to be unhappy as he was going to be a very important person to me in labour. In the end, he just came round through listening to other people who'd had their babies at home.'*

Making the decision to have a home birth can sometimes be difficult because of resistance from health professionals: *'I was surprised by my GP's negative attitude. He discussed the three local maternity units with me but stated quite categorically that he would not be happy for me to have a home birth.'*

Although attitudes towards home birth are changing amongst health professionals, some GPs and midwives still feel insecure when it comes to caring for a woman who wants to have her baby at home. After all, health professionals do most of their training in hospitals. Your doctor may explain to you that he or she feels unable to care for you if you want a home birth, but will be happy to refer you to a doctor or midwife who can: *'My GP said she was happy to care for me during my pregnancy and after the birth and that she would find another doctor from the practice who would cover me for a home birth.'*

'I'm lucky enough to live in an area where it is relatively easy to book a home birth. Although my GP chose not to be involved, he didn't try to dissuade me and left my antenatal care to the midwife. I was very happy with this arrangement. My midwife agreed to a home delivery even though I had had a forceps delivery with my first child. She was extremely positive about it all.'

Choosing a hospital birth

WOMEN WHO choose to have their babies in hospital find it comforting to know that there will be lots of midwives and doctors around; some feel that a technological birth is likely to be safer; some are attracted by the special facilities such as birthing pools which hospitals can offer (although it should also be said that it's quite possible to hire a birthing pool for use at a home birth):

'I chose a hospital because it was my first child. I'm not very brave and I would like as many people there as possible to help me. Having opted for the hospital, I wouldn't change it.'

'I wouldn't feel relaxed having a baby at home even if I knew I was having a full-term, healthy baby. I would like to be in a hospital and have all the professionals and all the equipment around me.'

'I decided quite early on that I wanted a hospital birth rather than a home birth. We wanted to minimise any risk. We made a joint decision. I didn't go to look round any of the hospitals; I just went for the one that was nearest.'

'I decided to go to the nearest hospital. Once you've seen the people there a few times, they seem quite human and that makes all the difference. Basically, I made the decision on gut reactions.'

'*I feel that things are* recommended *at the hospital, but are in no way forced on you. I'm very happy with that.*'

If you are thinking about giving birth in hospital, it is just as important as when choosing a home birth that both you and the person who will be your labour companion are happy about the decision: '*I wanted to go to hospital in case anything went wrong. My husband thought it would be best, too.*'

Choosing the Domino scheme

THE DOMINO SCHEME means, in theory, that one midwife looks after you throughout your pregnancy, goes into hospital with you for the delivery, and accompanies you home again a few hours afterwards. Although the scheme isn't available everywhere and in practice you may not have the same midwife with you in labour who looked after you during pregnancy, research suggests that it's a very popular

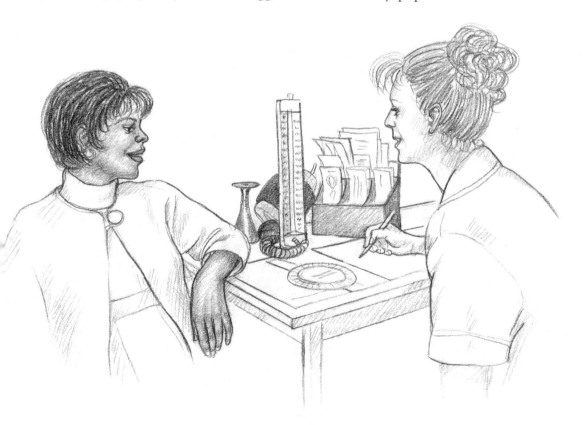

CHANGING CHILDBIRTH

The Winterton and Cumberlege Reports, 1992–1993

During the Parliamentary Session of 1991–1992, the Health Committee of the House of Commons conducted an investigation into Maternity Services in the United Kingdom. Under the chairmanship of Nicholas Winterton, MP, the Committee heard the views of midwives, obstetricians, paediatricians, GPs, health and social services administrators, dieticians and neonatal nurses. Most importantly, the Committee also listened to many women who spoke about their own experiences of the maternity services or who represented other women who had used or would use them in the future. Representatives of The National Childbirth Trust, the Maternity Alliance, the Association for Improvements in Maternity Services, the Stillbirth and Neonatal Death Society and the Society for Support after Termination for Abnormality spoke at length to the Committee about the kind of care they felt women wanted during pregnancy, when they were in labour and in the early days and months of parenthood. A 130-page summary of the Committee's findings was published at the beginning of 1992. It stressed repeatedly that health professionals should not presume to know what is best for any individual woman, but confine themselves to the task – a very important one – of providing information to help women make their own decisions about the kind of care they want. The Health Committee stated that midwives should be the key professionals to care for the vast majority of women who have perfectly normal pregnancies and births and that obstetricians should only look after the few women who have complicated pregnancies. The Committee decided there was no evidence to suggest that home birth is unsafe for healthy women and asked health professionals to ensure that every woman knows she has the right to choose to have her baby at home.

Following the publication of what became known as the Winterton Report, the Government set up an Expert Maternity Group to consider the Report's findings. This group was chaired by Baroness Julia Cumberlege and published its own Report in 1993 entitled *Changing Childbirth*. It is a much shorter document than the Winterton Report and far more readable; you should be able to see a copy of it at any central library. *Changing Childbirth* reinforces the recommendations of the Winterton Report and states that:

'The woman must be the focus of maternity care. She should be able to feel that she is in control of what is happening to her and able to make decisions about her care, based on her needs, having discussed matters fully with the professionals involved.'

The essence of *Changing Childbirth* is captured in the three 'Cs': Choice, Control and Continuity:

CHOICE: a woman should be able to choose the type of care which she feels is best for her (for example, home birth or hospital birth; to receive maternity care from midwives or doctors)

CONTROL: she should feel in control of what is happening to her because she is able to participate in decisions about her care

CONTINUITY: She should be able to get to know a small group of health professionals during her pregnancy who will care for her until a few weeks after her baby is born, rather than having to meet a different professional at every stage of her maternity care.

Changing Childbirth is an exciting and revolutionary document. It constitutes a Bill of Rights for childbearing women. Maternity services are now being planned in accordance with its recommendations and women should soon be able to have more say in their care than they have ever had before.

scheme with women. It gives them the satisfaction of developing an excellent relationship with one midwife whom they can confide in and whom they can trust to help them achieve the kind of birth they want. You may, however, have to be persistent if you want to choose a Domino delivery:

'When I first went to the doctor and said I wanted a Domino, he put on my booking form that he didn't think I was suitable, but when I saw the midwife, she said, "Of course you can, no problem."'

'I went to my booking appointment and I asked about a Domino. The midwife said that it was not a good idea because I was having my first baby and I'd be tired after the birth and it would be much better if I had a few days in hospital. However, I stuck to my guns and I'm glad that I did because my experience was that hospital isn't a very good place to recover. I recovered much better at home.'

'That's the good thing about the Domino system: you go in with the midwife when she thinks you're ready and then you're discharged within six hours. So you use the hospital and have your own midwife and get home quickly – ideal.'

Schemes very similar to Domino are likely to be available to more women in the future. This is because a recent government report, called *Changing Childbirth*, recommends that women should see just a few midwives for their maternity care. At present, it's quite likely that the midwife whom you see at your GP's surgery will not be the midwife who helps you give birth, or that, if you are going to the hospital for your antenatal checks, you see a different midwife and doctor every time you have an appointment. This makes it very difficult for the health professionals to get to know you and for you to get to know them. All over the country, the way in which midwives work is now being changed and soon, pregnant women should find themselves being looked after by a small team of midwives who will take responsibility for them from when they find out they are pregnant until after the birth of their babies. This will make it much easier for women to get information about their choices for birth, to ask questions and to feel relaxed with their carers. Perhaps it's never been such a good time to be pregnant!

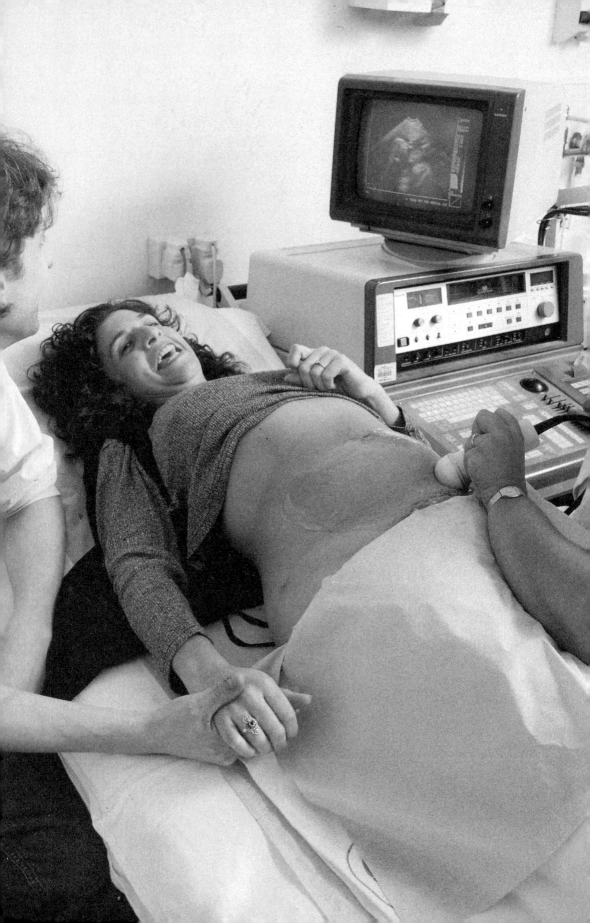

CHAPTER *three* *Antenatal testing*

EXPECTING A BABY was probably, in many ways, a very much easier business for our mothers and grandmothers than it is for women today. Our mothers were often not certain that they were pregnant until they had missed at least a couple of periods; today, it is possible to know within days of having sex whether or not you have become pregnant. This means that during the first three months of pregnancy when miscarriages are common, women are now fully aware that they are losing a baby whereas, in earlier days, they would either never have known they were pregnant, or not been sure.

Women today do not imagine that their babies might die unlike childbearing women a century ago who would quite definitely have anticipated this possibility. Because women now choose, for the most part, to have only one or two pregnancies, and many choose not to start a family until they are in their late twenties, thirties or even forties, it is really important that their few babies are healthy. On the back of women's and society's high expectations of childbearing, there has developed a whole range of antenatal tests which aim to detect whether an unborn baby has a problem such as spina bifida or Down's syndrome which is likely to affect him physically or mentally after birth.

These tests bring with them all sorts of decisions for the woman and her partner. The most difficult and heart-rending decision of all can be whether or not to end a pregnancy. But there are 'smaller', yet also very difficult decisions to consider such as which test carries least risk for the mother and her baby, at what stage in pregnancy it is best to have tests, and whether to have another test to confirm the results of a first test.

Understanding the concept of risk which is the foundation of antenatal screening tests is not easy. Screening tests do not tell you whether your baby definitely has a certain condition, but only how much at risk of having that condition he is. The mother confronted with a test report which states that her risk of carrying a Down's syndrome baby is 1 in 180 may find this result very difficult to grasp. 1 in 180 doesn't sound very high, but because it is a greater risk than the test's cut-off point of 1 in 250, she has been told that her blood test is 'screen positive' which sounds as though the risk is very real indeed. She may go on to ask herself what it might mean to her to have a baby with Down's syndrome or what it might mean to her to have a termination of pregnancy.

The decisions which need to be made about antenatal testing are, therefore, not trivial; they may well affect you, in one way or another, for the rest of your life. Getting support while you are making decisions about testing is, therefore, vital. You can choose to talk to your midwife, consultant, GP, partner, friends and other women who have been through the same tests. It's important to get as much information as you can; lots of women don't ask for information and look back and wonder why they made the choices they did.

ANTENATAL TESTING: SCREENING OR DIAGNOSTIC

It's really important to understand the difference between a SCREENING test and a DIAGNOSTIC test:

A **screening** test tells you whether you are at increased *risk* of having a baby with a particular condition such as Down's syndrome. It does **not** tell you whether your baby has Down's syndrome (or any other condition). To know for certain, you need to have a diagnostic test.

A **diagnostic** test tells you for certain whether your baby has certain serious conditions such as Down's syndrome or spina bifida.

GETTING INFORMATION

HOW MUCH information a pregnant woman is offered about the different tests she can have is variable. Sometimes finding out about a particular test is entirely dependent on chance: *'I picked up a magazine and read about CVS (chorionic villus sampling) and thought, "Gosh, that sounds better than an amniocentesis because it's so much earlier". I then asked to have it, but it was never suggested to me.'*

Other women find that health professionals spend a lot of time talking to them about tests: *'At the booking visit, my midwife talked through with me in some detail what our options were for testing and what we could do afterwards depending on the results. My GP also talked through the tests with me.'*

SOME OF THE CONDITIONS WHICH ANTENATAL TESTS DETECT

These are some of the conditions which are commonly associated with antenatal testing; there are other rarer conditions which can be picked up as well.

Down's Syndrome

This is a 'chromosomal abnormality' which means that there is something wrong with one of the genes which the baby inherited from his parents. It is the most common cause of severe mental disability in the UK. About 1,000 babies who have Down's syndrome are born each year.

Edward's Syndrome

This is also a chromosomal abnormality. Babies born with Edward's syndrome have small heads and often have a cleft palate. Their hearts and digestive systems are generally not properly formed. Most die in the first year of their lives.

Turner's Syndrome

All children born with Turner's syndrome are girls. They have a distinctive appearance, a little like a Down's baby, but are generally not mentally disabled. They tend to have heart problems and their reproductive organs do not develop properly.

Spina Bifida

This condition means that the vertebra of the baby's spine do not properly protect his spinal cord. Spina bifida can be very serious so that the person affected is paralysed and incontinent, or it may be much less serious and cause the person no problems at all during his life.

Anencephaly

The baby's brain and skull have not developed properly which means that the baby can only live for a few minutes or hours after his birth.

Cleft Lip and/or Palate

In the uterus, the baby's mouth develops in two parts which then join together. Sometimes, the parts do not join and the baby is born with a hole in his lip and/or the roof of his mouth. Surgery for these conditions is now excellent and cleft lips are treated as early as 3–4 months of age with cleft palates being closed during the second year of the baby's life.

'I asked my GP to refer me for a CVS test which she did. A few days later, I received a phone call from a midwife at the hospital who was responsible for counselling women about to have antenatal tests. We had a very long conversation in which we discussed the risk of losing the baby because of the tests, the risk of me carrying a Down's syndrome baby based on my age, what would happen if the result was positive for an abnormality, and how and when a termination could be performed. She also sent me written information.'

There are so many tests available now it is a good idea to sort out which tests, if any, you are going to have. Because the accuracy of nearly all of them depends on their being carried out at a specific point in pregnancy, it is important to organise them as soon as your pregnancy is confirmed: *'I saw my GP when I was 5 weeks pregnant specifically so that I could ask for early referral to the hospital and identify the "right" combination of tests and when to have them.'*

Either the mother or father of the child may have very strong feelings about testing as a result of what they have read or heard, previous experience, or their feelings about having a disabled child. While the couple may agree to let the views of one take precedence, it is still important that they do this only after considering all the available information:

'When I got pregnant, Matt said his first wife had had an amniocentesis because of her age and he was more or less insistent that I should and I just went along with it without even thinking what might happen if there was anything wrong. I wish I'd thought a bit more about it now.'

'We talked about not having the tests, but ultimately Reece went along with my decision because I'm the one who stays at home and although he would have to face the consequences of being the father of a disabled child, I would be the one who was doing most of the day-to-day care.'

Deciding not to have any tests

SOME WOMEN decide right at the beginning of their pregnancies that they are not going to have any tests at all. This may be because they wouldn't consider having an abortion even if there was something wrong with the baby, or because they consider the risks of the tests to be much higher than the risk of the baby being abnormal:

'I asked not to have the tests. In fact, my midwife assumed that I would. She asked me how old I was and then she said, "Well, I assume you'll be wanting the tests," and I said, "Well, no, I don't want to." And even after I'd said that, she then said when she was taking blood, "Shall I just take enough in case you decide that you do want the screening test?" There's a lot of pressure on you to have the test. The problem is I know that I couldn't do anything about a result that was abnormal; I know I couldn't have an abortion.'

'We've decided not to have any screening at all because a friend of ours had the Triple Test and came out with a 1 in 49 chance of having a Down's and when the baby was born, he was fine. But she'd had to go through all that trauma about whether or not to have an amniocentesis and whether or not she'd have an abortion, so we're not going to have any screening.'

The decision not to have testing may also be made because of earlier tragedies in the couple's life: 'I don't want any tests. I don't think I could have anything done if there was something wrong. Having lost two babies, I couldn't possibly abort this one.'

TESTS AVAILABLE

Chorionic villus sampling (CVS)

THE EARLIEST test which a woman can choose to have is CVS or chorionic villus sampling. For most women, the main attraction of this test is the fact that, should the result be abnormal, the pregnancy can be brought to an end at an early stage: 'I had CVS; I was very keen to have it. I actually asked to have it. I think I would have been offered it anyway because of my age. It's routine to offer it in my area to anyone who will be over 35 at the time of delivery, and I wanted to have it because you can have it earlier in pregnancy than an amniocentesis. I thought that if there was any problem and I did decide to go for a termination, at least it would be as early as possible. I had the test at 12 weeks.'

As with every aspect of the care she receives during pregnancy, in labour and after the birth of her baby, how the woman copes with antenatal testing depends to a very large extent on the support she

CHORIONIC VILLUS SAMPLING (CVS)

Type of test: DIAGNOSTIC

When is it done?
Around 11 weeks

What conditions is it looking for?
Down's syndrome
Turner's syndrome
Edward's syndrome
(*not* spina bifida)

How is it done?
The doctor passes a fine needle either through the wall of your abdomen, or into the vagina and through the cervix, and uses an ultrasound scan to help her find the placenta so that a very small piece of it may be sucked out through the needle. The procedure can be uncomfortable, but isn't normally painful. It takes from 10–20 minutes and is done in the out-patient clinic of your local hospital.

How long before the results come through?
7–10 days

If the result is abnormal, what next?
You could choose:
● To do nothing
● To have a termination of pregnancy (abortion).

receives: *'I was well counselled beforehand by a midwife and so it was quite a positive experience.'*

Fully understanding what is happening makes the procedure itself much more bearable: *'The procedure wasn't comfortable, but it wasn't as bad as I'd expected. I felt it was handled very well and I was given lots of information and I had the results within 48 hours; I was phoned at home.'*

Research shows that CVS is associated with more miscarriages than amniocentesis. Some women who are old enough to be at increased risk of having a Down's baby decide against the CVS test for this reason: *'I decided to have an amnio rather than CVS because of the risks involved. The hospital we're near seems to have fewer miscarriages after amnio than CVS – at least, that's what we were told.'*

There have been some reports that having CVS very early in pregnancy, before 11 weeks, may result in the baby's being born with abnormal arms and legs. Although CVS is now performed later than it used to be, some couples remain anxious that there may still be a risk of their baby being hurt by the test: *'We were offered CVS but told about the risk of miscarriage – 2%; the risk of the test being wrong – 2%, and, most important to us, the possibility it might damage the baby. We decided instead to opt for amniocentesis.'*

WHAT IS CLEAR from the different reasons which motivate women either to have or not to have CVS is that the decision is ultimately a very personal one. There are no absolute rights or wrongs about antenatal testing; the decision to have a test can only be based on what each individual woman sees as its advantages and disadvantages.

Blood tests

THE AFP TEST (which measures the level of alpha-feto-protein in a sample of the mother's blood), the Double Test (which measures the level of human chorionic gonadotrophin as well) and the Triple Test (which in addition measures oestriol levels) are all blood tests which assess the risk of the mother carrying a baby with Down's syndrome or spina bifida (and some other conditions). It is important for women to understand that these are screening tests and therefore not conclusive. The tests aim to give the woman an idea of how much at risk she is of having a baby with a disability. She can then use this

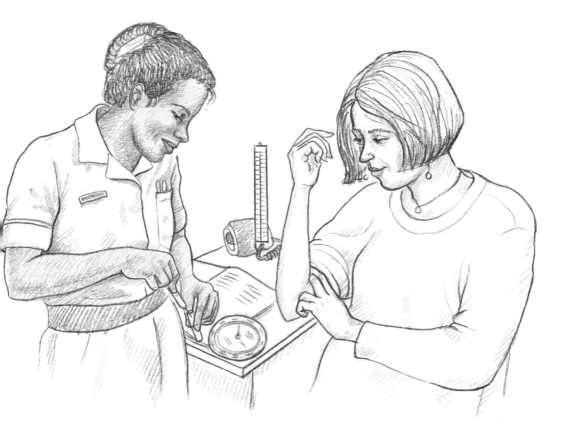

THE DOUBLE OR TRIPLE TEST

Type of test: SCREENING

When is it done?
15–18 weeks

What conditions is it looking for?
Down's syndrome
Spina bifida
Anencephaly
Turner's syndrome
Edward's syndrome
and some other rare conditions

How is it done?
By taking a small quantity of blood from your arm.

Although these tests used only to be available privately, many health authorities now provide them free of charge; some offer them to all pregnant women and some only to women over 30 or 35 who are at increased risk of having a Down's syndrome baby. If you are under 30 and want to have a test, *ask*, and you will almost certainly be able to have it.

The Triple Test looks at three different markers in the mother's blood to assess what the risk of her baby having Down's syndrome is; the Double Test looks at two different markers.

How long before the results come through?
48 hours

If the result is abnormal, what next?
You could choose:
● To do nothing
● To have a 'high resolution' ultrasound scan to check the baby's spine if your baby is thought to be at risk of spina bifida
● To have an amniocentesis.

information to make further decisions about testing:

'I had the Triple Test done privately and also booked myself in for an amniocentesis because I was over 37. The Triple Test results were good for my age so I cancelled the amniocentesis.'

'When I first went to the hospital, I was given a leaflet about the AFP Test. I decided that since there was no risk to the baby with the test, I might as well have it and depending on what the results were, I'd decide what to do next. And even if the result was positive, I might not do anything more because of the problem of it showing positive when the baby is all right.'

Even when the woman is at very low risk of having a baby with Down's syndrome or any other problem, and even when she has agreed to have the AFP test simply because it is on offer, waiting for the result can be nerve-racking: *'They said ten days until the result and you're counting the days and when ten days have gone, you start thinking it must be OK. You're sitting there during those ten days and every time the phone rings, you're thinking, "Well, I wonder if that's going to be the hospital?"'*

It is very common for the woman to be contacted only if the AFP result is abnormal: that is, either higher than average suggesting she may be at risk of carrying a baby with spina bifida, or lower than average suggesting that her baby may have Down's syndrome. She often hears nothing if the test is within normal limits. This can be very unsatisfactory: '*I think it would be nice to have a letter through the post telling you the result's normal; otherwise you're thinking, "Well, have they got my test mixed up with someone else's?" I'd like a letter in my hand to say the test's been done and it's OK.*'

Even after receiving the news of an abnormal result, it is a sad fact that some women find they have to endure more waiting until they are able to see a doctor with whom they can discuss what to do next: '*A midwife called at my home on Friday and told us there might be something wrong with the baby, but did nothing to inform us further. We were left to spend the weekend desperately trying to find out the implications of having a high AFP result. I went to the hospital on Monday morning and the midwife there told me I was at risk of having a spina bifida baby and that I must wait to see a doctor. Two hours later, I went in to see the doctor.*'

'*When I was 16 weeks pregnant, I had a Double Test. About two weeks later, my midwife phoned and said she had some bad news and that I needed to go to hospital the next day for an amniocentesis. I tried to question her but all she would add was that my baby was at risk of Down's syndrome and I could talk to a doctor at the hospital. Needless to say, I was distraught for 24 hours.*'

Some women live to regret having had the AFP test because an abnormal result puts a doubt in their minds as to whether or not the baby is healthy. If the baby is suspected of having spina bifida, it may be possible to choose to have a high resolution ultrasound scan to confirm the suspicion, rather than having to undergo an amniocentesis which carries a risk that the baby will miscarry. If the baby is suspected of having Down's amniocentesis is necessary to provide definite evidence one way or the other. Some women, however, do not want to choose amniocentesis because, if the result is positive, it leads immediately to a decision about terminating the pregnancy:

'*I was very upset when I got the bad news about the AFP and spent a sleepless night running through the options regarding amniocentesis and whether I'd have an abortion. I remembered vividly from my days as a nurse how really upsetting late terminations are and I knew that I would have to be very*

BLOOD TESTS FOR ANTENATAL SCREENING

Although a pregnant woman's blood can be tested to see whether her baby has any one of several conditions, it is mainly used to test for spina bifida and Down's syndrome.

Down's syndrome is the most common cause of serious mental disability. Young women are at lower risk of having a baby with Down's syndrome than older women. At the age of 20, your chance of having a baby with Down's is about 1:1700; at the age of 45, your chance is 1:30. Blood tests are used to give a more accurate assessment of risk than that based on your age alone. So you may be told that the risk of having a Down's baby at your age is 1:200 but the risk according to your blood test is 1:350. This means that you are at a much smaller risk of having a Down's syndrome baby than most women of your age. If, on the other hand, your risk according to your age is 1:500 but your risk according to your blood test is 1:60, you are at much higher risk of having a Down's baby than other women of your age. Most hospi-

tals use a cut-off point of a risk of 1:250 which means that if your risk is less than 1:250, your blood test will be described as 'screen negative' and if your risk is greater than 1:250, your test will be described as 'screen positive'. So, the fact that your test is screen negative doesn't mean for certain that your baby does not have Down's syndrome, and the fact that you are screen positive doesn't mean that your baby does have Down's syndrome.

The risk of a baby having spina bifida is not related to the mother's age. It can however be related to where she lives; more babies are born with spina bifida in some parts of the UK than in others, namely the North West, Wales, Scotland and Northern Ireland. Overall, about 4 in every 1000 babies born have spina bifida, but it's important to remember that spina bifida doesn't have to be serious. Some children with spina bifida have hardly any problems, while others will need to be in a wheelchair and require care 24 hours a day.

AFP (Alpha-Feto-Protein)

Type of test: SCREENING

When is it done?
15–18 weeks

What conditions is it looking for?
Spina bifida
Down's syndrome
Turner's syndrome

How is it done?
By taking a small quantity of blood from your arm

How long before the results come through?
About 10 days (often women are only told if the result is abnormal)

If the result is abnormal, what next?
You could choose:
● To do nothing
● To have a 'high resolution' ultrasound scan to check the baby's spine if your baby is thought to be at risk of spina bifida
● To have an amniocentesis.

convinced of the baby having a serious abnormality before I could endure one. I wished I'd never had the AFP test but I hadn't considered the full implications beforehand.'

A blood test which comes back as 'screen positive' and states the woman's risk of having a baby with Down's syndrome can be very hard to understand: *'If you know that you have a baby with Down's syndrome, that's very different from being told you've got a 1 in 48 chance of having one.'*

THE INITIAL DECISION to have a screening test now leads to another about whether to have an amniocentesis. This test can tell conclusively if the baby is affected with Down's syndrome or other serious problems. But it can be an uncomfortable procedure for the woman, risky for the baby, and means three weeks of waiting for the result. If the result comes back positive, another decision is immediately required – whether to carry out a termination of pregnancy. It can seem, therefore, that the nature of antenatal testing is for small decisions to lead to ever harder ones having to be made.

Amniocentesis

SOME WOMEN choose not to have any blood tests but simply to opt straight away for an amniocentesis: *'I didn't really trust the AFP because I've come across people where the result has been normal and they've had Down's syndrome or spina bifida children. So I requested to have an amnio. It's been very reassuring for me. The results take quite a while but I wasn't too stressed during that period because I didn't consider myself at particularly high risk, so I didn't mind waiting.'*

A fear of the extra responsibilities which come with having a Down's syndrome baby drives some women to choose amniocentesis even though they know the test could cause a miscarriage: *'I was prepared to have an amniocentesis because I felt that if I had a Down's child, that would be the end of my life, my work, and my marriage probably, and I didn't want to have one because I've seen two or three people with Down's children whose lives have fallen apart.'*

AMNIOCENTESIS

Type of test: DIAGNOSTIC

When is it done?
16–18 weeks
(but the test may soon be offered much earlier in pregnancy)

What conditions is it looking for?
Down's syndrome
Edward's syndrome
Turner's syndrome
Spina bifida
Anencephaly
and other rare conditions

How is it done?
A fine needle is put through the wall of your abdomen and using ultrasound to guide her, the doctor takes a sample of the amniotic fluid (waters) which surround the baby. This fluid contains cells from the baby and these are sent to a laboratory. The procedure takes from 10–20 minutes to carry out and is done at the local hospital in the out-patient department.

How long before the results come through?
3–4 weeks

If the test is positive, what next?
You could choose:
● To do nothing
● To have a termination of pregnancy (abortion).

A health professional's view of a woman's risk of having a Down's baby may be very different from her own: *'My GP quoted a percentage risk of Down's for my age group – I think she said 1 in 300 – and said that in her view, this was not significant. I didn't entirely agree. So I decided to go ahead and ask for amniocentesis.'*

There may be pressure put on the woman to state that she will definitely have a termination of pregnancy if the amniocentesis result is positive. While some women have no doubt that they would choose to end the pregnancy if their baby were diagnosed as having Down's syndrome, others simply want to know for certain so that they can have time to prepare themselves for the birth of a baby with a disability: *'I was told that an amniocentesis could only be performed if I would make the decision in advance to terminate if the results were positive. It was only my argument that I wanted to know if I was having a baby with Down's syndrome so that I could make adequate preparation for its arrival that enabled me to have the amnio without making a decision about termination.'*

Some women resist the pressure to discuss a termination in advance of the amniocentesis by appearing to go along with the wishes of the hospital while reserving judgement: *'My obstetrician made it clear that it was worth me having an amniocentesis provided that we would go for a termination. And I said, "Fine", although I hadn't really decided; I reserved judgement to decide later and say, "Sorry, I'm going ahead with my pregnancy."'*

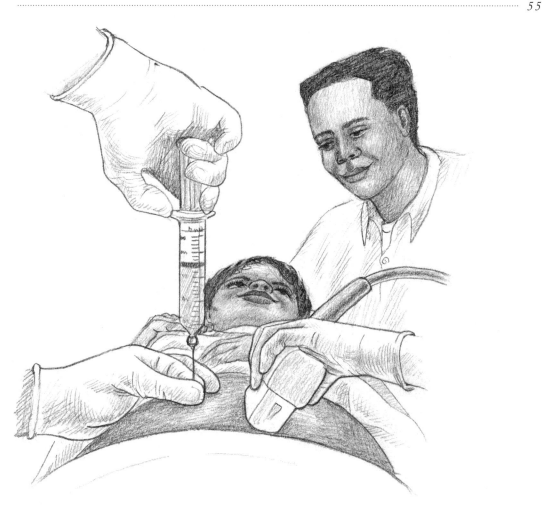

There should be no pressure on the woman one way or the other to make a decision in advance of knowing the results: *'I chose not to consider the termination question before the amnio. The consultant reacted well and said it was a "philosophical attitude".'*

Having the amniocentesis performed can be a very different experience for different women. The difference may in part depend on how worried the woman is about the outcome: *'I wanted to have amniocentesis for total reassurance; I'm not at high risk of having a Down's baby because I'm only 27. The amnio was OK; it wasn't painful or anything – I just felt a push as the needle went in.'*

PROS AND CONS OF ANTENATAL TESTS		
Test	**Pros**	**Cons**
CVS (chorionic villus sampling)	Carried out early in pregnancy A termination, if needed, is simple to perform and probably easier for the mother to cope with psychologically because it is done so early in pregnancy.	Risk of miscarriage – the likelihood of this will depend in part on the skill of the person carrying out the test. Ask your hospital about its rate of miscarriage following CVS (probably about 2%) May not be available at your local hospital.
Alpha-Feto-Protein	A simple blood test which carries no risk to the baby	Fairly unreliable – for example, most of those women told they are at high risk – 19 out of 20 – will NOT have a baby with spina bifida.
Double Test/Triple Test	A simple blood test which carries no risk to the baby	Can be very hard to know whether to have more tests if your risk comes back as higher than average. After all, even a 1 in 5 risk of having a Down's syndrome baby still means that you are far more likely not to have an affected baby.
Amniocentesis	Gives you a definite result	Risk of miscarriage afterwards; ask your hospital what its rate is (probably 1–2%) Carried out fairly late in pregnancy (16–18 weeks) You have to wait 3 or 4 weeks for the result If you decide on a termination, you will be well on in pregnancy and will have to go through labour.

PROS AND CONS OF ANTENATAL TESTS		
Test	**Pros**	**Cons**
Ultrasound scans	Can give all sorts of information about the health of the baby You can see your baby on the screen Can be carried out at any point in pregnancy	The usefulness of the scan will depend on (a) how good the radiographer is at interpreting the scan (b) how good the scanning equipment is (c) how long you are scanned for There is a shortage of long-term research into ultrasound; it may have effects on unborn babies which we don't yet know of.

'I was almost 36 when I conceived and my husband and I had already discussed having an amniocentesis. Damian was with me throughout the test. I wasn't really expecting to feel as shocked as I did afterwards; the feeling of contraction as the needle goes in and comes out was very strange although I had been told to expect it. I was told to rest for 24 hours afterwards – I think I was in a state of shock for at least a day.'

The procedure for taking two samples of fluid in a twin pregnancy can be more complicated and time–consuming: *'They extracted the fluid from around the first baby with no problem, but there was a membrane in the way of the second and they couldn't get any. I was there several hours with a few rests along the way. In the end, they had to call in the senior man who finally did it. But I had had the needle inserted in several places across my belly.'*

Although the likelihood of miscarriage is small after an amniocentesis, the risk is there. There are occasions when antenatal testing leads to a series of events which change the woman's life for ever: *'I was not given any counselling about the AFP test which I accepted as routine. I was twenty weeks pregnant when I was told that, although I was only 26, I had the risk of a woman of 37 of having a Down's baby. The amnio was booked for the next day, so I had no time at all to think it over and in any case, I was on my own and in a state of extreme anxiety. I had the amnio on Tuesday and the following Friday, I started getting pains which I now know were the beginning of labour. I was admitted to hospital that night and gave birth to a little girl six hours later. I was not informed of the results of the amnio until I rang up the hospital and was told that the baby had been normal. This was all nearly four years ago and I am still mourning the loss of my daughter who would have been just about ready to go to school now had it not been for the antenatal testing.'*

Waiting for the results of an amniocentesis may take up to four weeks and the time can seem endless when so much may depend on the outcome: *'If the result had been positive, then my GP would've arrived unannounced on the doorstep, so for at least the last week of the three weeks' wait, I was a gibbering idiot every time someone knocked on the door.'*

A negative result can bring with it tremendous reassurance and allow the woman to relax and enjoy the remainder of her pregnancy. Strangely, however, it doesn't always have this effect:

'My friend had AFP which was slightly low and then she had an amniocentesis and everything was fine and normal, but she still couldn't stop worrying. It didn't reassure her; she spent the rest of her pregnancy worrying, so for her it didn't work.'

'Having an amnio and then waiting for the results changed my whole attitude towards the baby and the last few months of my pregnancy were very frightening because I was so worried even after I'd had the negative result. I'm now planning my second pregnancy and I really don't know whether to have any tests this time.'

A positive result leads to the necessity of considering whether to end the pregnancy. While some women feel quite strongly prior to the amniocentesis that they would have an abortion if Down's syndrome was diagnosed, they may find themselves uncertain when it comes to finally making the decision: *'The baby's got Down's syndrome, but I don't know how badly the baby might be affected. It could be quite a mild case.'*

The influence of other people can be paramount: *'We had a friend whose daughter had spina bifida and she died when she was twelve and he said to me one day last year: "If my wife and I had known, we would not have had her. Although we loved her, she had no life at all." And that's made a very strong impression on me.'*

IN ALL CASES where a woman is thinking about terminating her pregnancy, it is essential that she receives sympathetic counselling from health professionals. She can also choose to turn to other women who have had to make the same decision, to a minister, to organisations which help parents facing a termination or which can help them understand what is involved in looking after a disabled child:

'I contacted the Down's syndrome Association who sent me through their standard literature. In addition, I contacted the local University which is involved with the Down's syndrome Association and went to see their work with children and families with Down's babies.'

If a woman has a twin pregnancy and one baby is found to be normal, but the other to have Down's syndrome, it is possible to carry out what is called 'selective termination' and abort just one baby:

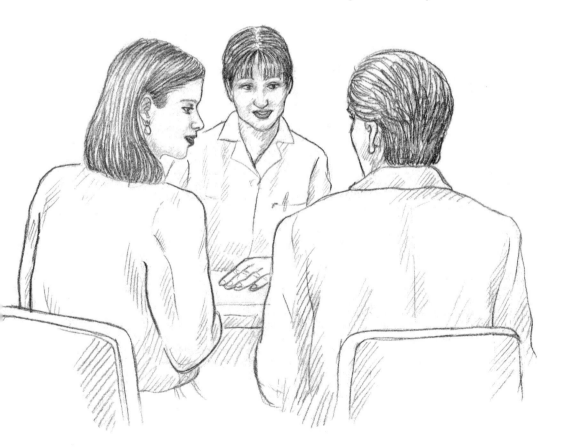

'The consultant was extremely kind and courteous and talked to us and gave us lots of time. There was a small risk of miscarriage but we knew without question that we wanted to go ahead. We had to put our faith in him and his high reputation. But I couldn't help thinking that night, "What if they get the wrong baby?" We went back the following day for the termination. The baby's heart was injected and it was instantaneous and afterwards, they immediately showed me the other baby moving about and obviously unaffected. I was very upset. I had to sweat it out for three more days until they phoned me with the results of a blood sample they had taken from the aborted baby to say that yes, the baby had got Down's. For the rest of my pregnancy, I needed constant reassurance about the other baby.'

The decision not to abort may be made on moral or religious grounds or because the woman doesn't believe that having a disabled baby is necessarily a terrible thing or because she wants to know and care for her baby however briefly. A midwife remembers a couple who chose to have their baby in spite of the unlikelihood of it surviving: *'The amniocentesis came back that the baby had something really serious and they decided not to abort and they carried on to have a normal labour and yes, the baby was clearly not going to survive. But they got to hold the baby and the baby died in her arms. She felt that this was how it should be and they could actually give the baby the comfort of their arms and get something back themselves.'*

Ultrasound scanning

WHEN ULTRASOUND scanning in pregnancy was first introduced in the United States, there was so much excitement amongst both women and their doctors that scans were being carried out, in some cases, weekly, throughout pregnancy. Since those early days, more restraint has been exercised so that now, in this country, routine scanning generally takes the form of two scans only, one to date the pregnancy at about 12 weeks and one to look for abnormalities in the baby at about 18 weeks. Some well-informed people, both lay and professional, are beginning to urge even greater caution in the use of scanning, warning that very little long-term research has been done into its possible effects on children. One Norwegian study suggested that scanning led to an increase in the number of left-handed children and speculated that this might be due to changes in the development of the brain brought about by ultrasound.

As with all the other forms of testing discussed above, women have different views about ultrasound and are entitled to make up their own minds: *'I thought the scan was wonderful – the baby looked as if it was moving around.'*

'It's helped the baby to have an identity for me – and certainly for my partner.'

'It's almost as if the technology is there, so we'll use it. I don't agree with that.'

Some are alarmed by recent unfavourable television and newspaper reports about ultrasound scanning in pregnancy and become very confused about what to do: *'Every time I read something about the dangers of ultrasound, I read something which says the total opposite. Nothing's been proved. It's very hard to make a decision.'*

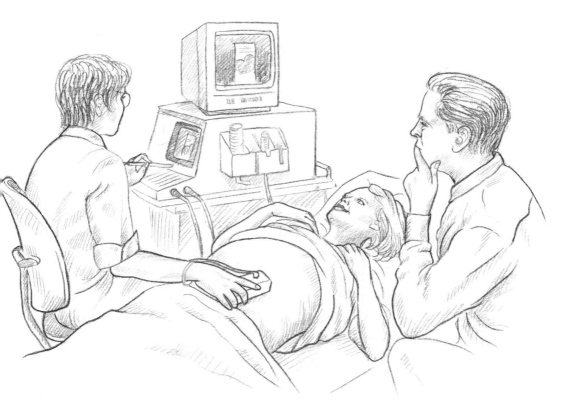

ULTRASOUND SCANNING IN PREGNANCY

Nuchal Test

Type of test: SCREENING

When is it done?
10–13 weeks (only on offer at a few specialist centres)

What condition is it looking for?
Down's syndrome

How is it done?
You have an ultrasound scan and the radiographer or doctor measures the amount of fluid beneath the skin behind the baby's neck. This measurement can indicate the possibility of the baby having Down's syndrome.

How long before the results come through?
Immediately

If the test is positive, what next?
You could choose:
- To do nothing
- To have CVS (chorionic villus sampling)
- To have a blood test (AFP or the Double or Triple Test)
- To have amniocentesis.

Fetal Anomaly Scan

Type of Test: SCREENING

When is it done?
18–20 weeks

What conditions is it looking for?
A large range of abnormalities: the scan checks the baby's arms and legs, spine, heart, brain and kidneys
Spina bifida
Anencephaly
Cleft lip and palate

How is it done?
A cold jelly-like substance is put on your abdomen before the radiographer passes a transducer across your abdomen and looks at the picture of the baby on a screen. You will be able to see the image too and the radiographer will point out your baby's face, hands and feet.

How long before the results come through?
Immediately

If the scan shows an abnormality, what next?
You could choose:
- To do nothing
- To have another more detailed scan
- To have amniocentesis.

A high resolution ultrasound scan which is an extremely detailed scan using a very expensive scanner could pick up spina bifida in a baby. In this case, ultrasound becomes a diagnostic test rather than a screening test.

Women can find themselves under a lot of pressure to conform to the routine care provided by the hospital: *'And they were coming along and they were almost being abusive in the end because I would not have an ultrasound. I kept saying, "I'm sorry, I will not have one. I do not want to have one. This is my body and my decision. I've weighed up all the pros and cons and I do not want an ultrasound." And they were saying, "The doctor's getting very upset because you won't." The emotional blackmail was amazing.'*

If the baby is seen on the screen during an early scan, a miscarriage can be even harder to cope with: *'It almost made it harder seeing that Lydia was OK, moving around and the heartbeat and everything and then losing her five weeks later.'*

On the other hand, the image provided by the ultrasound may become part of the healing process following a miscarriage: *'In some ways, although it upset me seeing the baby on scan and then his dying, at least I saw him and it made him real. Seeing him on the scan, we have a lasting picture and that's all we've got. So that's really important.'*

INFORMED CHOICE

THE PRESSURES created by antenatal testing are immense. The decisions which have to be made about whether to have a certain test and then about what to do should the test be positive are very complex indeed. They are decisions which can only, in the last resort, be made by the woman herself. Women's feelings about testing are extremely varied and what will be the right decision for one woman will not be so for another. Finding your way through the maze of tests is not easy but as with all other aspects of pregnancy care, it seems that the most satisfying decisions are reached when the woman feels that she has been fully informed. If the woman knows what options she has and has been helped to think about what she will do if test results are positive, and if she has been given time to make her decision and has not been pressurised, the likelihood is that she will feel content about whatever tests she decides to choose:

'I felt that the midwife gave me all the information I needed at the time to make a decision. She stressed that whatever I decided, I could change my

WHAT HAPPENS AFTER A BLOOD TEST

Rhesus factor

Some women are described as having Rhesus negative blood. This can be a problem if the baby has Rhesus positive blood. During delivery, blood cells from the baby can pass into the mother's bloodstream and the mother reacts to the foreign blood cells by manufacturing antibodies to destroy them. If the mother becomes pregnant again with a Rhesus positive baby, these antibodies will pass to the baby and start to destroy his red blood cells.

So after giving birth, every Rhesus negative mother is given an injection of anti-D. This masks any of the baby's red blood cells which have got into her bloodstream, so that the mother does not manufacture antibodies against them.

Women who are Rhesus negative have their blood tested repeatedly during pregnancy to make sure that they are not forming antibodies. If antibodies are found, the baby can be treated with blood transfusions while still in the uterus.

Nowadays, Rhesus negative women don't have problems if they have proper antenatal care during each of their pregnancies.

Rubella testing

If your blood sample shows that you have no immunity to rubella:

1. You will be advised to keep well away from any child or adult thought to have rubella (sometimes called German measles)

2. It will be suggested that you are vaccinated against rubella once your baby has been born (you then need to avoid getting pregnant for the next three months)

3. If your blood sample shows that you have been recently infected with rubella, you will be offered a termination of your pregnancy (abortion). This is because there is a very high risk of the baby being born with serious problems.

Anaemia

If your blood tests shows that you have low levels of haemoglobin, you may:

1. Be advised to eat more foods such as bread, cereals and potatoes which are rich in iron; more fruit and vegetables which contain vitamin C and therefore help your body to absorb iron

2. Be prescribed iron tablets (which, for maximum effect, should be taken with the first and last meal of the day).

All pregnant women appear to be slightly anaemic because their blood is thinner than that of non-pregnant women (ie the same amount of red blood cells but much more diluted). Nowadays, there is a strong feeling that mild anaemia during pregnancy should not be treated as thinner blood probably improves the circulation through the placenta.

TESTING FOR HIV (AIDS)

Some Health Authorities are routinely testing the blood of all pregnant women for HIV, but the testing is anonymous ie the result cannot be traced back to you. The test should not be done without your consent. If you want to know whether this is happening, ask the midwife or doctor who takes blood from you at your booking visit.

If you specifically want to consider having an HIV test, ask to discuss the matter with a counsellor, your midwife or doctor. All hospitals should provide counselling from someone with training on HIV issues. You need to think carefully about the pros and cons before having a test.

mind. I later saw her again and discussed my decision and she gave me a date for the test and told me what would happen and how I would be informed about the result. She also gave me a telephone number if I wanted any more information. I feel that the counselling helped me to make an informed decision.'

BLOOD TESTS IN PREGNANCY

When you 'book' at the antenatal clinic the midwife will take some blood from your arm for routine testing:

1. To find out your blood group
2. To find out whether you are Rhesus negative
3. To assess your haemoglobin level (whether you're anaemic)
4. To test for syphilis (sexually transmitted disease)
5. To assess your immunity to rubella (German measles)
6. To test for blood problems such as sickle cell disease which is common amongst West Indian people, and thalassaemia which is common amongst Mediterranean people

Blood samples for haemoglobin testing are taken again at:
28 weeks and 36 weeks of pregnancy

If you are Rhesus negative, you may have further blood tests at:
28, 32, 36 and 40 weeks of pregnancy

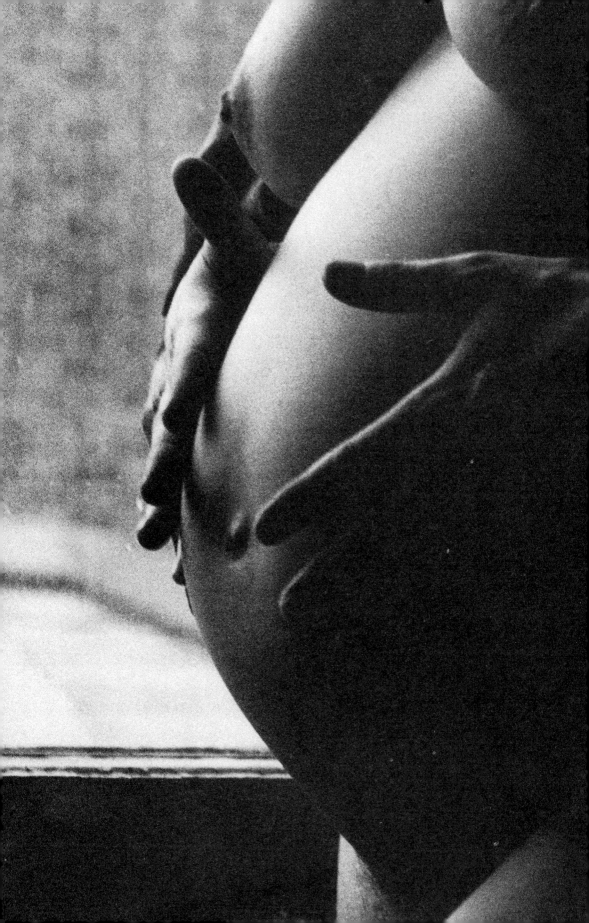

CHAPTER *four* *What labour is like*

HOWEVER MANY WOMEN you talk to about what happened to them during their labour and what labour felt like to them, one thing is absolutely certain: your experience will be quite different from any of theirs. This is not to say that you can't learn a lot about birth from listening to other mothers. Certain things happen in all normal labours: contractions or labour pains open up the neck of the womb until it is as wide as is necessary for the baby to pass through – usually about ten centimetres; then the womb and the mother together push the baby out into the world, and finally the placenta or afterbirth is delivered. But even within this basic framework, there are many variations and it would be unwise to presume that because you have read all the books and been to lots of classes that you know exactly what is going to happen to you.

FEELING IN CONTROL

MANY PREGNANT women talk about how important it will be for them to feel in control of their labour. Nonetheless, there may be parts of your labour when you feel very out of control, when the contractions are extremely strong and powerful and you feel taken over by them. There may be moments when the birth of your baby seems infinitely far off

THE THREE STAGES OF LABOUR

Labour is divided into three stages:

The First Stage

This is when contractions make the cervix or neck of the womb open up from 0 to about 10 cms. Your progress in first stage is assessed according to how many centimetres your cervix is 'dilated'. If you are having your first baby, first stage usually lasts from about 12 to 18 hours.

The Second Stage

This is the 'pushing' or 'expulsive' part of labour when you give birth to your baby. It generally lasts about two hours for a first baby.

The Third Stage

After the baby has been born, the placenta needs to come out of the uterus and this happens in the third stage of labour. Third stage can last a few minutes or over an hour (see third stage box).

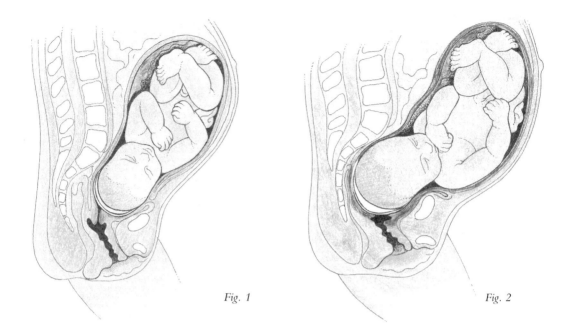

Fig. 1

Fig. 2

Figures 1 – 4 show how the cervix (the neck of the womb) opens during the first stage of labour. The baby moves lower into the mother's pelvis whilst his head turns so that his face is towards her spine. This is the position in which it is easiest for him to be born. You can see how the bag of waters bulges down in front of the baby's head towards the end of the first stage (Fig. 4). The waters generally break now. When the cervix is open as wide as it needs to be for the baby to come

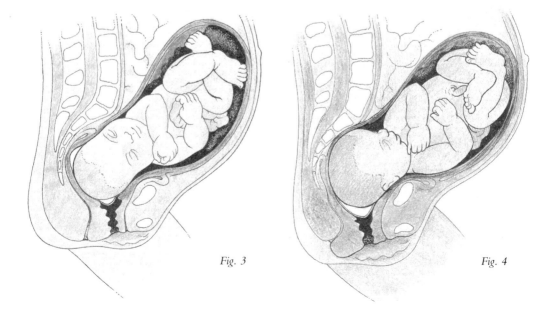

Fig. 3

Fig. 4

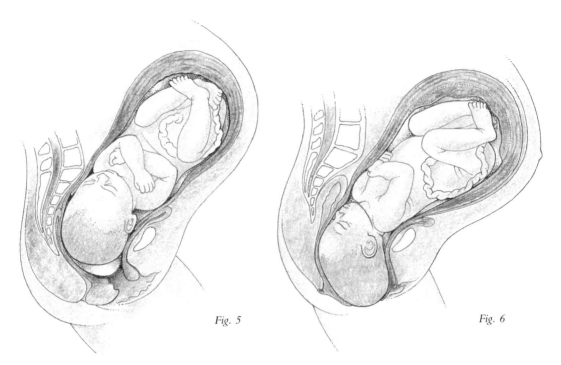

Fig. 5

Fig. 6

through (about 10 cms.) the uterus and the mother together push the baby out of the pelvis (Figs. 5 – 7). The baby is working hard to be born as well, now untucking his head and stretching his neck so that he can move round the mother's pubic bone and out of the vagina. After his head has been born, the baby turns his head so as to help bring his shoulders out of the vagina (Fig. 8) and his whole body will be born with the next contraction.

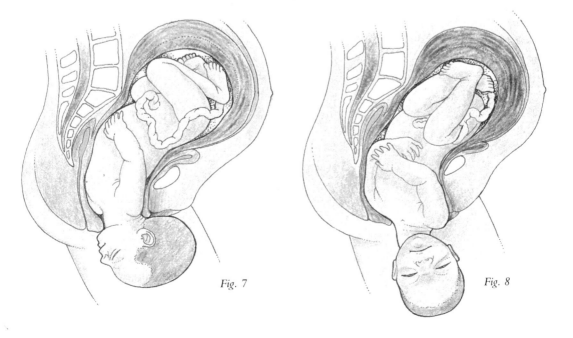

Fig. 7

Fig. 8

and you feel that you will never get to that magical moment when he is finally placed in your arms. It's difficult to feel in control at these points. What will help you is understanding what's going on, knowing how far on in labour you are and whether your baby is okay. If your contractions are coming so fast that you can't ask for information yourself, your labour supporter can ask for you and then pass the information on to you. Often labour supporters are better than health professionals at communicating with women in strong labour because they know them so well.

Feeling in control has little to do with not shouting or swearing or throwing your nightie off because you're too hot! It's about your midwife and labour supporter talking to you, keeping you informed, encouraging and reassuring you. Not being communicated with leads to feelings of panic: *'The more they were rushing around and not telling me what was going on, the more I was panicking. They kept telling my husband to go out of the room and he didn't know what was going on either. He was very frightened.'*

When communication has been good in labour, most women feel satisfied with their care no matter what course the events of labour have taken: *'Because the midwives had given me such confidence in myself and listened to what I wanted, I really had faith in my own body and I felt that it was doing what it was meant to do. I'm glad that I've experienced labour.'*

The start of labour

ONE OF the things women and their partners are often very anxious about during pregnancy is how they will know when labour has started. It's helpful to understand that labour doesn't have a definite starting point. You're not pregnant one minute and then in labour the next, as if moving from one physical state to a completely different one. The neck of the uterus, the cervix, changes over a period of days in the early part of labour. From being long and firm like the tip of the nose, it becomes shorter and softer so that it is more like the texture of the lips. You may be quite unaware that anything is happening. Or you may have several days of niggly, period-like pains when you begin to sense that labour is getting underway. Eventually, it is

AM I IN LABOUR?

● *You have had a 'show'*

This means that the small plug of mucus which sealed the neck of the uterus (cervix) during pregnancy has dropped out indicating that the cervix is starting to soften and open. It's a very early sign of labour and you need to stay calm and wait for something else.

WHAT'S OKAY

The show is jelly-like and slightly pinkish because it is streaked with a little blood.

WHAT'S NOT OKAY

The show should not be accompanied by a sudden loss of blood similar to your period. If you are losing blood freely, contact your midwife, GP or the hospital straight away.

● *Your waters have broken*

Ring the midwife who is going to help you give birth at home, or the hospital if you are going to give birth there and ask for advice. You will be asked the following questions:

● When do you think your waters broke?
● Did they go with a gush or did you simply notice that your underwear was damp?
● What colour is the fluid you are losing?
● What does it smell like?
● Have you had a show?
● Are you having any contractions?

WHAT'S OKAY

The waters are clear or straw-coloured.

WHAT'S NOT OKAY

They should not be greeny-brown in colour, or foul smelling. If they are muddy, this probably means that your baby has opened his bowels in the uterus which is often (although not always) a sign that he is distressed and perhaps needs to be born quickly.

● *You are having contractions*

Contractions may be the first sign you have that your labour has started – women don't always notice that they've had a show and the waters don't break, in the majority of cases, until labour is well underway. It can be very difficult to know from the contractions how far on in labour you are, especially if this is your first baby. Ask yourself the following questions and contact your midwife if you are unsure about what to do.

ASK YOURSELF:

● When did the contractions begin?
● How long are they lasting now?
● How frequently are they coming?
● How painful are they?
    (difficult to answer – but ask yourself whether you can still talk or work while having one, or whether you need to stop and lean onto something and concentrate on your breathing)
● Am I happy coping on my own or with my labour supporter?
● Would I prefer to have my midwife with me?

If the answer to the last question is 'yes', phone your midwife and ask her to come to you if you are having a home birth or Domino delivery, or go to the hospital where you are booked after letting the labour ward know when you will be arriving.

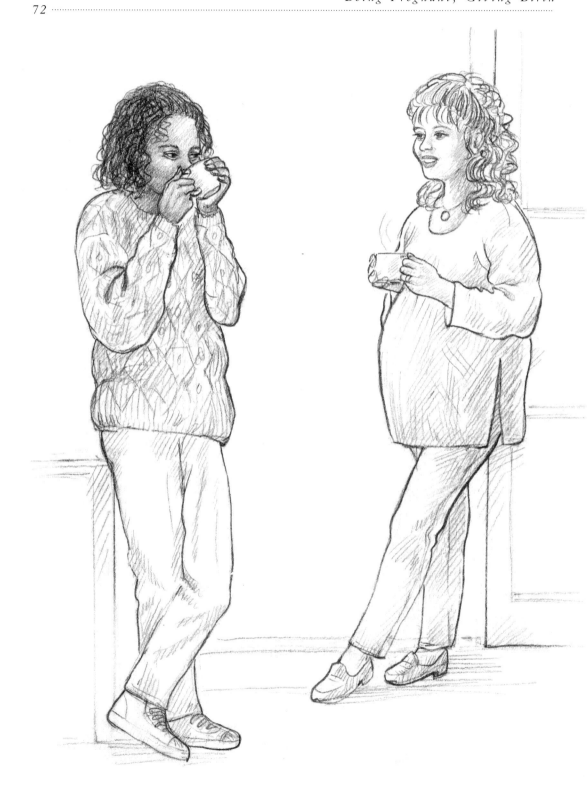

obvious that your baby is coming; there may be a show when the plug of mucus which has sealed the cervix during pregnancy drops out, or the waters break or the contractions begin to make themselves plainly felt:

'I had a show as I got out of the bath; it was very obvious. I just knew straight away that that must be what it was.'

'I'd had a few days of what I thought were Braxton-Hicks contractions, coming few and far between, and then I was lying in bed, reading a book, and I heard this "pop" and my waters broke and there was quite a lot which surprised me.'

'I had invited a friend to come round for the afternoon and while we were talking, I began to have contractions. I knew they were the real thing even though they didn't hurt much and I could go on talking to Melanie while I was having them. In fact, I didn't tell her I had started in labour and I walked all the way to the car park with her, contracting every ten minutes.'

Labour gets underway gradually as the amount of oxytocin, the hormone which causes contractions, builds up in your body. Contractions don't start 'out of the blue'. Ever since you were a baby yourself, growing in your mother's womb, your uterus has been contracting. If the baby you are pregnant with is a little girl, her womb is contracting inside you, too. All through your life, your womb has continued contracting but you haven't been aware of it except if you've suffered from painful period cramps. During your pregnancy, you may have been surprised that, on occasion, your bump goes very hard, like a stone. This is your womb contracting, getting ready for labour. Pregnancy contractions are called Braxton-Hicks contractions; not every woman feels them and it doesn't matter if you don't. As labour gets under way, the contractions of the uterus become gradually longer and stronger and, unlike Braxton-Hicks contractions, they come at regular intervals. Some women first notice their labour pains when they are coming at perhaps five minute intervals and the contractions remain at this level throughout their labours. Others become aware that labour has started when they are having two or three contractions an hour, and then as labour progresses, find

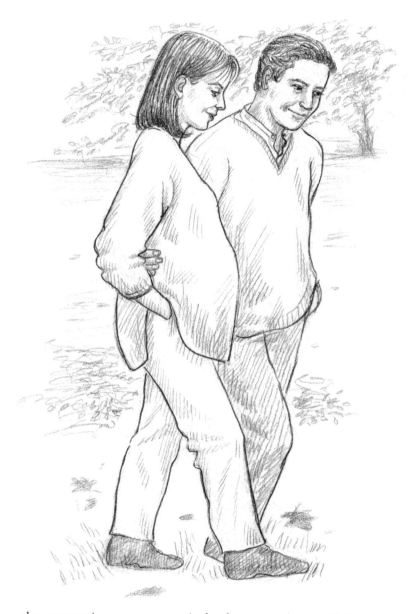

the contractions get progressively closer together until they are coming every two minutes.

   While you are at home before you go to the hospital or before you
call the midwife, it's a good idea to continue your normal routine as
much as possible: *'I ate a light lunch and kept myself busy around the house
until mid-afternoon when I could no longer focus on anything else except what
was happening in my body.'*

EATING AND DRINKING DURING LABOUR

For many years, health professionals told women that they should not eat or drink anything other than water once they had gone into labour. Hospitals were very strict about this; the fear was that if the mother needed to have a caesarean section because something went wrong during labour, the food in her stomach, or rather the acid used to digest it, might pass into her lungs while she was unconscious under a general anaesthetic. What we now know is that when you fast, the amount of acid in your stomach does not decrease but increases. Some hospitals still don't allow labouring women to eat, but give them antacids every four hours to neutralise the acid in their stomachs. Antacids are actually much less effective in neutralising stomach acid than are small quantities of food taken at regular intervals.

You may hear it said that you should not eat in labour because food will take a very long time to digest. The thing which really slows down digestion in labour is having pethidine for pain relief, and you are probably much safer to have light snacks in labour and not have pethidine than to have pethidine and starve. Many midwives and doctors now feel that telling a woman she can't have anything to eat in labour is a mistake.

The arguments for eating in labour are:

- Women in labour are engaged in hard, physical work and need food for energy and to avoid exhaustion. Eating during labour may well make contractions and the whole birth process more efficient

- When you have not eaten for a long time, you feel weak, bad-tempered and unable to cope. Exactly the same applies to women in labour

- Research carried out in America has shown that women who are allowed to eat during labour have fewer forceps and ventouse deliveries and fewer caesareans; they feel happier about their labours and have healthier babies.

Food is a major part of our enjoyment of life and essential to keep us alive. Even the great religions of the world which dictate that people should fast at certain times make an exception for pregnant women!

Decide how you feel about eating in labour and have a talk to your midwife about what she thinks. Together you can probably come to an agreement.

'Barry and I settled down to watch videos with me leaning on a huge pile of floor cushions. Within about an hour, things seemed to go up a gear. The contractions became stronger, more intense, longer and quite regular. During each one, I buried my head in the pillows and groaned to myself. When the contraction was over, I went back to watching the video.'

It's not unusual to find that as soon as you arrive at the hospital or telephone for the midwife to come to you at home, contractions stop. Even though you were convinced you were in strong labour, the contractions simply disappear: *'I didn't realise that my contractions could just stop for no apparent reason.'*

'On Monday, I started to get quite strong contractions, every 5–6 minutes, for about two hours and so I called the midwives. As soon as they arrived, it all stopped. I went to bed and had a good sleep.'

Moving from your home to the strange environment of the hospital, or acknowledging that your labour is definitely underway by asking the midwife to come to you, is quite a big step. If you are very excited about your labour, very anxious and 'up-tight', your body will respond by making lots of adrenalin which is the hormone of 'fright and flight'. The adrenalin works against the oxytocin which is making your womb contract and so the contractions stop. This is really a very clever device on nature's part. Nature presumes that if you are frightened, you and your baby must be in danger. It is therefore logical to have a way of stopping labour until you are no longer frightened and feel safe enough to give birth to your baby. Once you have settled into the delivery room at the hospital or welcomed the midwife into your house and she has unpacked her things, you will start to relax and feel more secure. Soon contractions will get going again and your labour will continue.

What contractions are like

WHEN WOMEN are having normal labours without any medical interventions, and when they have people with them who are well known to them and who understand and can respond to their needs, the pain of labour is generally manageable. Contractions are like waves; waves build up gradually, gaining in strength all the time, until they reach a crest when they crash down and race towards the shore, losing their power and finally trickling away into nothing on the beach. When the wave is finished, there is a slight pause before the next one begins: *'It's bearable because it's not continuous pain. You get a space in between.'*

Contractions start as small waves which become bigger and stronger as labour progresses. Generally, the woman has time to adjust herself to the increasing strength of her labour: *'It doesn't come suddenly; it's a build up and if you can deal with it mentally and not get too tense, then you can get through the later stages. You can learn as you go along how to cope with things.'*

'You get used to it; your body helps you to.'

Contractions in the first part of labour can be felt in various parts of the body, but surprisingly, they're rarely felt at the front where the bump is:

'I felt the contractions in my back – really intense – not where I thought I would feel them.'

'The contractions were in my groin; it really hurt.'

'The contractions were down in my bottom, very low down.'

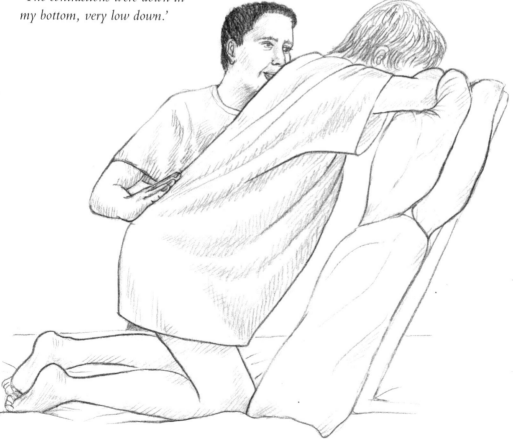

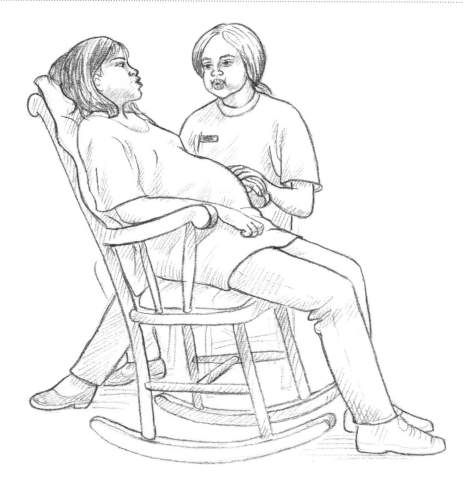

When the baby is being pushed out into the world during the second part of labour, the mother feels the contractions differently: *'The contractions were like shitting a brick. A very, very hard object. I remember thinking that while I was pushing!'*

Despite the pain of contractions, women can still find labour an exhilarating event: *'All the time, there's excitement underneath.'*

How labour progresses

IN THE early part of labour, women often find that they are restless and will try all sorts of ways of making themselves more comfortable: *'It was getting harder to cope and I was very restless. I kept going to the toilet, trying to vomit, and rocking myself madly during contractions.'*

It's impossible to say how long a first labour will last – anything from a couple of hours to a couple of days: *'It was short and incredibly intense. There wasn't time to think about it or get my act together. It was just happening. The contractions came like a tidal wave.'*

'Mine was a long labour, a forty-five hour marathon. I had lots of time to think. I even baked a pie during the first stage! What I mainly remember is being incredibly tired as I didn't sleep for two nights.'

Second time round, it's likely that labour will be shorter than it was the first time – but there's no guarantee: *'My second labour was precisely twice the length of my first. It lasted eighteen hours, but until the end bit, I think it was easier than my first.'*

Many women find that they are unaware of the passing of time and that hours slip by without their realising: *'I lost all sense of time from one morning to the next. I don't remember much about some of the labour.'*

At the end of first stage, when contractions are often coming fast and furious and are intense and painful, women may feel that they can't cope any longer. This part of labour is sometimes called 'transition': *'I kept saying, "I want to go home! I want to go home!" I'd really had enough.'*

'When I look back on it, I think I had quite a positive labour apart from the last half hour before I started pushing. This was the only point when I said, "Just give me an epidural; I can't take any more."'

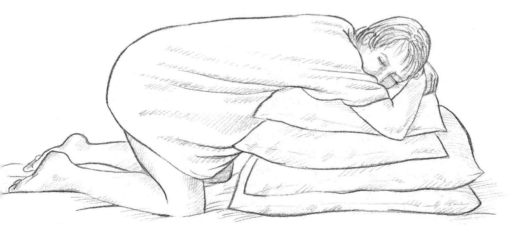

TRANSITION

At the end of the first stage of labour, when the cervix is almost fully open, women often experience a range of symptoms which mark the transition between the first and second stages of labour. Symptoms include:

- Shaking
- Suddenly feeling very cold
- Icy feet
- Hiccuping
- Being sick
- Feeling very weepy and helpless and wanting to give up
- Feeling very angry with everyone, including the baby, because labour hurts so much
- Being bad-tempered and abusive.

It's just that labour is hard work at this point and women feel that they can't cope any longer. What is needed is lots and lots of encouragement from your midwife and labour supporter, and reassurance that what you are experiencing means that very soon you will be ready to push your baby out into the world and hold him for the first time.

Don't worry – very few women experience all the symptoms outlined above, and some have none of them! After transition, it is common for the contractions to stop altogether for ten or twenty minutes, allowing the mother time to rest and renew her energy ready for pushing. Nature is not lacking in compassion!

Feeling that you want to push before the cervix is fully open

If you start feeling that you want to push and your midwife tells you that your cervix is not quite ready to let the baby come through, you can try the following strategies to control the pushing urge:

- Kneel on the bed or on the floor with your face on the mattress and your bottom in the air; this position will reduce the pushing sensation
- Try panting – three short pants and one long blow, saying to yourself: 'I . . . will . . . not . . . push'

The knee–chest position can help a woman cope with an early urge to push

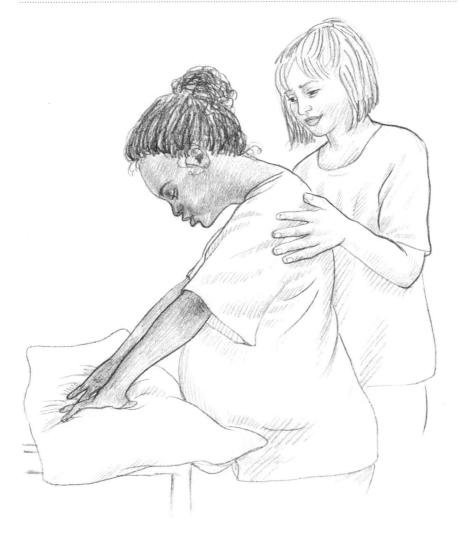

'My transition was very long and I stamped around shouting at the midwives, "Can none of you suggest something to do; I can't think any more!"'

Your uterus is working incredibly hard during this part of labour to open up your cervix fully so that your baby can come through and be born. Your labour supporter and midwife are also likely to be working hard, doing everything they can to make you more comfortable. Whilst you are completely wrapped up in contractions, transition may be a very anxious and emotional time for your supporter, especially if this person is your partner. He is probably feeling fairly helpless, wondering what he can possibly do to help you further, and worried in case what is happening is not normal and you and the baby are in danger. He may also be having to cope with some not very complimentary comments from you – women have been known to abuse their partners roundly at this point in labour!

Staying positive while you are going through transition, particularly if you are feeling sick and shivery and bad-tempered is very difficult, but everything that is happening is a sign that your labour is moving on rapidly towards the time when the baby will be born. After transition comes the second stage of labour when your womb starts to push your baby out into the world.

Giving birth

ONCE THE midwife has told you that the second stage of labour has started, you will probably feel much more hopeful again and ready to help your uterus push. In the first stage of labour, you may have felt that you were simply enduring the contractions, but in the second stage, you can participate actively in your labour and this can be very satisfying:

'I just wanted to push and when you get that feeling, the pain just seems to disappear; it changes.'

'Pushing felt completely instinctive – as if some kind of animal energy was taking over in me.'

However, the second stage can also be intense and frightening; the sensations which women experience are often much stronger than those of first stage and women use powerful words to describe how they felt:

'The baby's head moving down was very frightening as I really felt that I would split open.'

'I had an awful stinging sensation when the head was being born. I remember thinking, "I can't deliver this baby"; it was very painful and it was frightening to push and get the pain again.'

Some women don't get any urge to push but still try to push or are told to push even though their bodies aren't telling them that they should. This can make labour distressing and extremely hard work: *'The labour itself was only five hours, but my contractions had gone off by second stage and I had two hours of hell trying to push the baby out with no urge to push.'*

It's very helpful to remember that your uterus is more than sufficiently powerful to get your baby born without you doing any pushing. If you don't want to push, tell your midwife and listen to what your body is saying to you. Perhaps it would be helpful to try another position; perhaps it would be best simply to breathe deeply, following

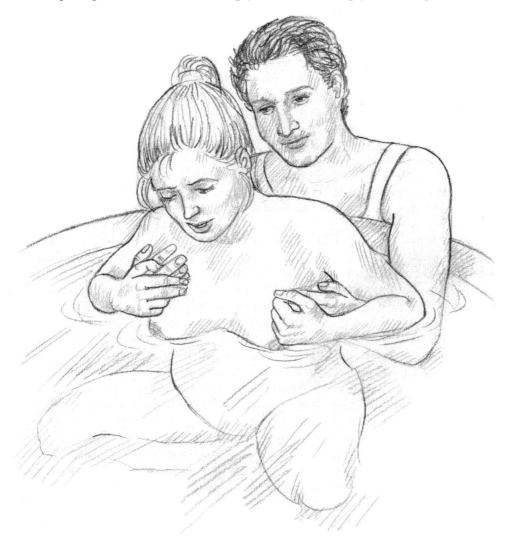

your breath right down between your legs in order to help your baby be born. Some childbirth educators feel it's better if women don't push during second stage so that birth can be a very gentle experience for their babies.

Labour is often a noisy experience, especially during second stage. But the grunts which the woman makes are helpful to her and part of the huge effort of giving birth. They also give important clues to the midwife about what is happening: *'I made a lot of noise in second stage.*

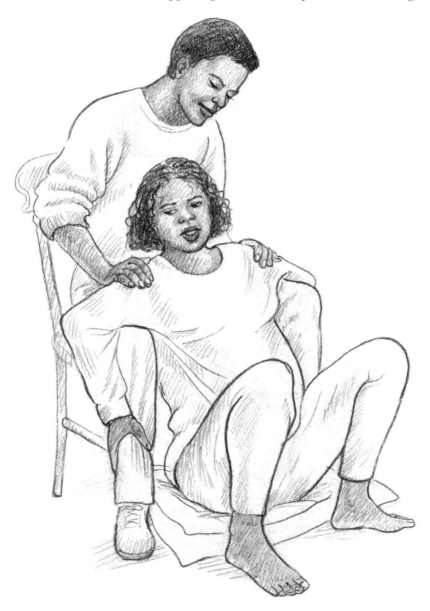

My midwife used the noises I was making to know where I was. She didn't examine me; she was marvellous.'

'I began to get the urge to push. I was aware of making a lot of noise at this point, but it was a wonderful way of releasing the intense pressure.'

Very fast labours

OCCASIONALLY, WOMEN find that they are in second stage almost before they have realised they are in labour. Babies who are born unexpectedly at home or on the way to the hospital sometimes come very easily. The mother in the following extract crouched down with her chest on the floor and her bottom in the air to try and give her husband time to get her to the hospital for the birth: *'It was about half an hour's drive to the hospital and my waters broke and I wanted to push when we were about half way there. I was on my hands and knees on the back seat of the car with my bottom in the air, trying not to push, defying the force of gravity. We got to the hospital and the midwife said to me, "What stage are you at?" and I was down on the floor with my bottom in the air, saying, "I want to push!" and she said, "Don't be silly; come into this room and give me a specimen of urine." And I thought, "You're joking; I want to have a baby!" She examined me and said I could push as the head was there. So I got up and squatted and just pushed and he was out and he was a 9lb 14oz baby and it was a very pleasurable experience.'*

The moment of birth

SOME WOMEN choose to lift their babies out of their bodies them-selves, and take them straight into their arms for the first cuddle: *'The baby's head eased out with the next contraction. It was such a relief to see this little dark head between my legs. We had to wait a couple of minutes for the next contraction before the rest of her body was born. As she came out, I put down my hands and lifted her onto me.'*

For other women the moment of birth is equally joyous but a differ-ent kind of experience because they are having a caesarean section: *'I heard a gush as my waters broke and I felt a tugging sensation inside me. Then the doctor shouted: "It's really big, it's a really big boy!" She lifted him above the screen so that I could see him. He was then placed face down on my chest. He started to suck immediately. It was the most satisfying experience of my life.'*

Twin births are different again: *'Suddenly the room was full of people. Everyone wants to see twins being born! My legs were in stirrups because the first baby was breech and I was having forceps. The registrar gave me some local anaesthetic, and then it was all pushing and pulling – pushing on my part and pulling on his. I felt a twang as the baby's legs came out. The doctor held her up for a moment so that we could see her and then she was whisked away to be checked. I wanted to push again and Joshua arrived face up. The midwife placed him on my tummy. He looked exactly like my other two boys. Then they gave me Anna. There I was with my legs still in the air and my arms full of babies!'*

Sadly, the moment of birth is not always the big event which the woman has been looking forward to. Some pain-killing drugs can make women feel so dopey that they hardly realise they have given birth, or for other women their baby may need the immediate

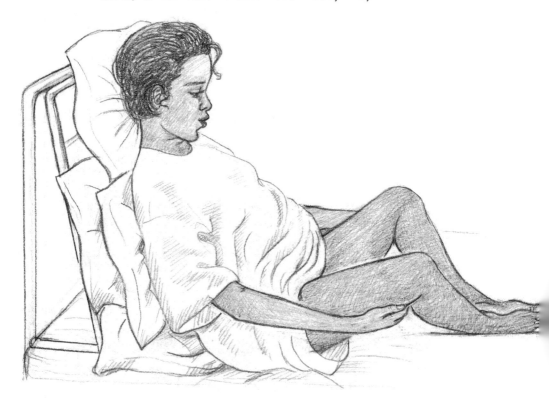

attention of doctors and be taken away to the Special Care Unit. This can lead to a feeling of having been denied something very important: *'My partner held him which I liked, but it's all so vague and I feel really sad that I can't remember much about it.'*

'I wasn't allowed to hold the baby. The midwife took him away and I didn't see him again for an hour. It felt very strange when he was brought to me – as if he wasn't really mine.'

Some women are simply too exhausted both physically and emotionally to be able to take charge of the baby immediately: *'I was very tired and they said, "We'll take him to the nursery and give him some milk" and I said, "Fine." I wanted to go to sleep. I was shattered.'*

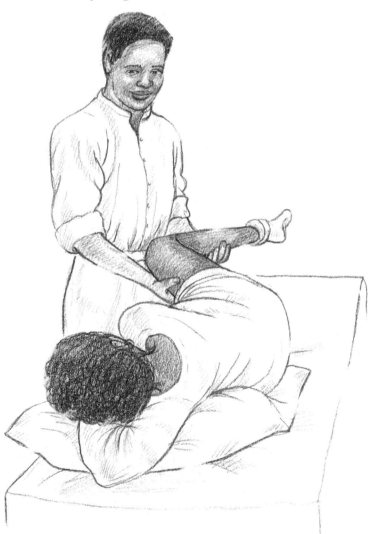

The baby may look very unlike what you were expecting. Some babies are purple when they are born, and some look grey and lifeless which is frightening. In a surprisingly short period of time, they turn pink and look quite different: *'He cried and I knew he was alive. He looked like a grey lump of clay and they gave him some oxygen. Then he cried again and turned pink and they wrapped him up in a green sheet. I asked if I could pick him up. I haven't really put him down since.'*

THIRD STAGE OF LABOUR

The third stage of labour is when contractions push the placenta or afterbirth out of the uterus. These contractions are generally not painful. There are two ways in which the third stage of labour can happen:

'Managed' third stage

- As your baby's shoulders are being born, you are given an injection in your thigh of a drug called syntometrine
- As soon as your baby is born, his umbilical cord is clamped in two places and cut in between so that he is now no longer attached to you
- The syntometrine makes your uterus contract very strongly to force the placenta out

- The midwife pulls on the cord which is still attached to the placenta inside you in order to help the placenta out
- The placenta is delivered within 5 to 7 minutes of the birth of your baby.

'Natural' third stage

- When your baby is born, his umbilical cord is not clamped
- You put your baby to the breast and encourage him to suckle. This stimulates your body to produce more oxytocin to make your uterus contract and push the placenta out
- The midwife waits and observes
- The time from the birth of your baby to the delivery of the placenta could be anything from ten minutes to an hour and a half.

THE PLACENTA AND AFTERBIRTH

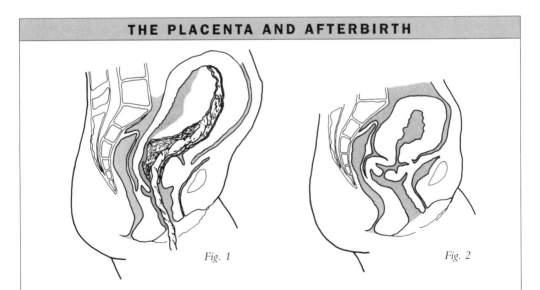

Fig. 1

Fig. 2

The placenta or afterbirth comes away from the wall of the uterus after the baby has been born and drops down into the lower part of the womb to be pushed out by the mother or helped out by the midwife (figure 1). The womb then contracts down (figure 2).

NATURAL THIRD STAGE

Advantages

Nature is allowed to take its course.

When your baby is born, he has two sources of oxygen – he is still receiving oxygen from you along his umbilical cord because it hasn't been clamped and he is starting to breathe for himself.

Your baby gets exactly the amount of blood nature intended him to have as the umbilical cord goes on pulsing for up to 10 minutes after his birth.

Disadvantages

You can only have a Natural Third Stage if you have had a natural labour – no pain-killing drugs (except for gas and air which is okay) no epidural, and no drip to stimulate contractions – and so long as you have been upright and mobile for most of your labour.

Third stage may take a long time.

You may lose more blood than if you had had syntometrine.

MANAGED THIRD STAGE

Advantages

Third stage is over very quickly.

Women are at risk of bleeding heavily in the third stage of labour. The injection you are given is to control bleeding. At the moment, research suggests that women who have the injection do bleed less than women who don't.

Disadvantages

Because your baby's umbilical cord is clamped as soon as he is born, he is no longer getting oxygen from you and must breathe immediately on his own.

Clamping the cord means that there is blood left in the cord which would normally have passed to the baby.

If the cord isn't clamped, blood rushes along it rather like a tidal wave when the syntometrine makes your uterus contract. This sudden deluge of blood may not be a problem for a healthy baby, but a baby who is not strong could find it hard to cope with.

Syntometrine closes up the cervix so if for some reason the placenta doesn't deliver within seven minutes, it will be trapped inside the womb and you will need to have it taken out in theatre. This is called 'a retained placenta'. 3–5% of women have this problem.

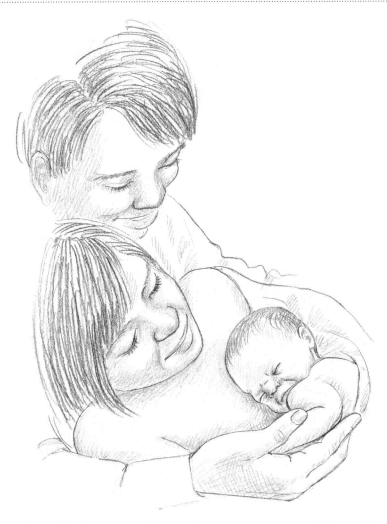

Just as labour often involves harder work than you have ever done before, and you feel the strongest physical sensations you have ever experienced, so the moment of birth can be charged with over-whelming emotion: *'I said, "Oh! Oh! It's a boy! It's a boy!" and I started crying and Peter started crying."'*

The arrival of the baby helps put the events of labour into perspective:

'Whatever you go through, once you see the baby at the end, you forget it, don't you?'

'I just couldn't believe that I'd got a baby and that everything was okay.'

Some women feel so empowered by labour, so strong and confident that they are ready to do it all over again! They have a feeling of immense pride in what they have achieved:

'It had been a long labour and I was exhausted, but I had a tremendous feeling of achievement. I had succeeded in giving birth!'

'I'd have another baby tomorrow! It's just the most amazing experience.'

TIPS FROM WOMEN WHO HAVE GIVEN BIRTH

WOMEN WHO have just had babies themselves are often the best source of good advice on how to prepare for labour and how to cope when it happens:

'It's really important to be well-prepared, so that you understand what's going on. Go to classes and read plenty.'

'I think you need to know all your options for pain relief beforehand because at the time, you can't rationalise what's on offer. It's better to have looked into it from the beginning.'

'If you're worried about something, ask and they will tell you.'

'Relax and let nature take its course; as long as you have people there to help you who know what's going on, there's nothing to worry about.'

'Your body tells you a lot of what to do.'

'Remember that it's only one day in your life and the baby's.'

And finally, you have to recognise that:

'Nothing can totally prepare you!'

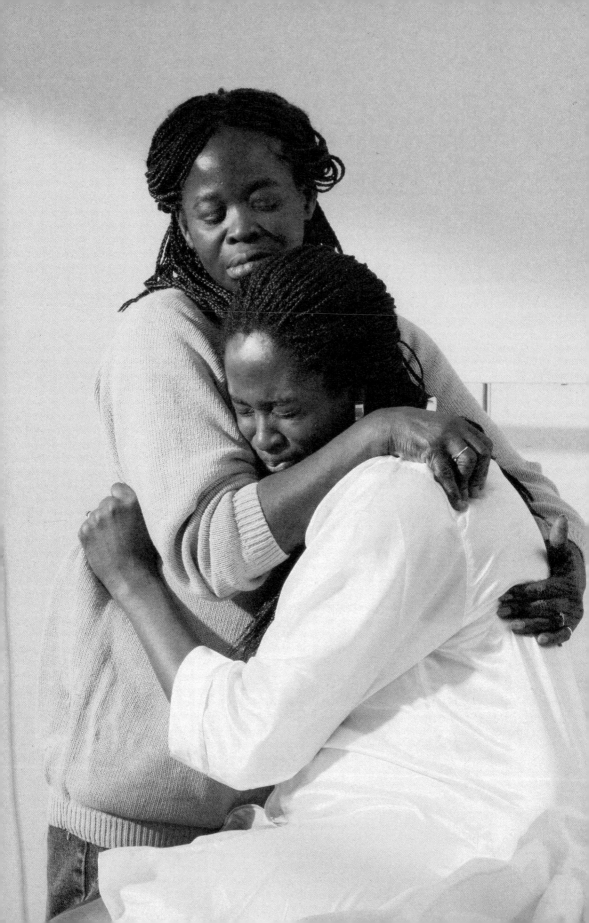

CHAPTER five

Coping with pain in labour

WORRYING ABOUT PAIN

PROBABLY THE vast majority of pregnant women are anxious about the pain of labour. What will it be like? How bad will it be? Will they be able to cope? The media present us regularly with images of labour which suggest that it is long, excruciating and often dangerous. Women who have already given birth can sometimes be unhelpful to others who are pregnant when they tell them horror stories about their own labours (stories which are, it has to be said, often rather exaggerated in the telling). When pregnant women go to their ante-natal classes, they find that their teacher spends a lot of time discussing pain in labour, suggesting practical ways of coping and offering infor-mation about the various drugs and medical procedures which are available for pain relief. Some women become so frightened simply anticipating the pain they may be going to feel that the last months of their pregnancies can be spoiled:

'I know that my body's capable but I'm frightened. They say that if you're frightened, your body tenses up and then you feel more pain and it all becomes a vicious circle. I'm frightened of getting into that and not being able to get out of it. I try not to think about when I go into labour because the more I think about it, the more frightened I get.'

'I've tried not to listen to people's horror stories – there is so much fear around. It's difficult to break through that and remain confident.'

'I buy all the baby magazines and when I was about three months pregnant, there was one article which was called "Everything You Need to Know about Stitches" and it went into really graphic detail about all the things that could go wrong. I just sat there in tears because I was so worried about the labour.'

...G WITH A
...HE LABOUR'

If ...is lying with his back against your ba... what your midwife describes as 'a posterior position') you may find that you have a lot of backache during your labour. The backache comes not just with the contractions, but continues in between them making it very difficult for you to rest and relax and prepare yourself to meet the next contraction. There are a number of things which might help you:

● Try getting down on all fours during contractions so that your baby drops away from your spine; this will help relieve the pressure on your back

● Your labour supporter or midwife can wrap a hot water bottle in a towel and place it in the small of your back; alternatively, you may find something very cold helps the ache, such as an ice-cold bottle wrapped in a towel

● Firm, continuous massage to the lower part of your back may be comforting. Your labour supporter can try placing the heel of his hand firmly against your tail bone and moving it round in small, firm circles. If you don't like this, say so!

● Encourage your baby to move round by making as much room in your pelvis as possible – keep moving; try squatting for a while which opens up the pelvis to its maximum capacity, and rock your hips in circles and from side to side.

Yet there is so much that you can do to help yourself in labour. Women frequently underestimate their own resources for coping with pain, and old wives' tales always emphasise the difficult parts of labour rather than the exciting and satisfying aspects. It would certainly be more helpful to the little girls who will one day be mothers if adults started to give them a different picture of labour from the traditional frightening one.

HOW THE PAIN HELPS

THE FIRST thing to say about pain in labour is that some women do not have any. These women may be few in number, but, you will also meet others, in addition to them who consider that the pain of labour was nothing extraordinary and very much within the range of what they had previously experienced in their everyday lives:

'I didn't experience any pain. I wouldn't call it pain at all. I'm not saying it was comfortable; it was definitely uncomfortable and I was very aware that it was all happening, but it wasn't painful and I was very much up and arguing!'

'I experienced quite intense period pains which weren't pleasant but I didn't experience pain in any frightening sense.'

In fact, not feeling pain in labour can be a problem when women are expecting that part of the transition to motherhood will be to go through a painful labour.

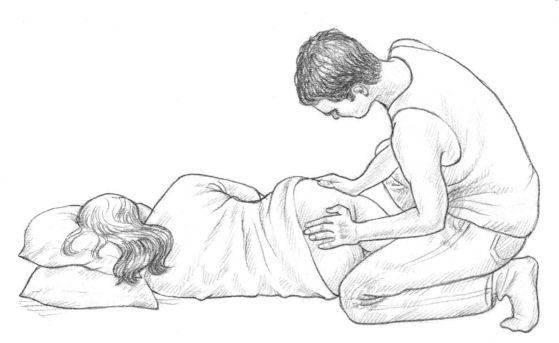

Women sometimes feel that the pain of labour is important psychologically because it's a test of their commitment to the baby:

*'I did feel that I had contractions but they weren't overwhelming and I really
miss that; I think I should have had that. So next time, I'm looking forward
to having some pain!'*

*'More and more I feel that the pain of labour is necessary. Not that I enjoyed
it — well, I did in some ways and for me, a pain-free labour isn't desirable —
no sense of achievement.'*

It seems unlikely, from an evolutionary point of view, that the pain of
labour should be beyond what most women can bear. Nature intends
the pain to serve some very important purposes. The first painful
contractions tell the mother that she is in labour; if mothers felt nothing at all, babies would run the risk of being born in some very
unsuitable places! The gradually increasing strength of contractions
gives the mother an indication of how far on in labour she is so that
as the time approaches for her baby to be born, she can summon help
and go to a safe place to give birth.

In everyday life, we respond in instinctive ways to pain. If you bang

HELPING YOURSELF COPE WITH PAIN

Getting Comfortable

The most important thing is to *get comfortable*! Whether you are having your baby at home or in hospital, move around all the time trying new positions to see which is best for you. The chances are that what makes you most comfortable will also make it easiest for your baby to be born. Nearly all women find that being upright in labour helps them cope better with the pain. This is because the bones of your pelvis can open up wider than if you are sitting on your tailbone, and because gravity helps your baby to move down through your pelvis. When the uterus contracts, it rears forwards and you will probably find it comfortable to lean forward yourself, so helping the uterus to work effectively.

There are all sorts of positions you can try – the only guide is what works best for you.

● Standing, leaning forwards onto a table, the back of a chair, a bed or your labour supporter
● Kneeling, leaning onto the seat of a chair, or onto your labour supporter's knees if he is sitting, or onto a bean bag or pile of pillows
● On all fours with your head dropped down
● Sitting 'cowboy fashion' astride a chair, leaning onto a pillow placed across the back of the chair
● Lying (if you are really tired and want to lie down) on your left side with a pillow between your legs
● Squatting supporting yourself by leaning forward onto your hands, or onto your partner's knees while he is sitting.

You will find many of these positions even more helpful if you combine them with rocking your hips forwards and backwards or round in circles. Rocking has been a form of comfort since time immemorial; you will find it soothing and it helps your baby to explore your pelvis and find the easiest way through.

Making a Noise

Don't hesitate! Don't feel that you shouldn't, that it's not the right thing to do, or that you will be considered a nuisance or a wimp. It is well known that making a noise is an effective form of pain relief – look at the way small children react when they're hurt. Labour is a noisy experience – if it helps you to groan or shout or make funny grunting noises, then do so.

Massage

When you hit yourself against something, your immediate reaction is to rub the spot which has been hurt. Rubbing causes the body to release natural pain-killing substances called endorphins. Massage is only a more sophisticated form of rubbing. Many women find having the lower part of their back massaged during labour is very helpful. Some like a lot of pressure applied to their tailbone in order to counteract the strength of contractions. Some don't want to be touched at all during contractions, preferring not to be disturbed; some like to be massaged in between contractions to help them relax. Tell your labour supporter or midwife where you want to be massaged and when; say what is helpful and what is not. Massage may be nicer if your supporter uses an unscented oil or your favourite massage oil on his hands to prevent friction building up when he rubs your skin.

HELPING YOURSELF COPE WITH PAIN

Breathing

Women breathe in all sorts of different ways during labour. Some take long slow breaths to carry them through the contractions; some lift their breathing over their contractions, taking small, shallow breaths; some breathe in steps, taking a small breath in, then another, and then a small breath out and another. As long as your breathing is even and doesn't become panicky so that you start gasping and end up feeling dizzy, sick and tingly, you're OK. It's generally helpful to concentrate on the out breath (you are programmed to breathe in!) but sometimes the out breath can be held back. So think 'out' when breathing and let your tension flow away as you breathe out.

Using Water

Most of us find that having a bath or shower when we are stressed is relaxing. Water is very soothing for aching muscles. The same is true in labour. Lying immersed in warm water helps many women relax and cope well with their contractions. If the water is deep enough, you will be able to use different positions to increase your comfort. If you haven't got the use of a birthing pool or bath, try taking a shower during labour instead.

Relaxation

All the things described above will help you relax, and if you can relax, you are conserving your energy and ensuring a good supply of oxygen to your baby (who is also going through labour too, don't forget). Having a good relationship with your midwife so that you feel free to ask her questions will also help you relax. Your labour supporter can use his first-hand knowledge of what helps you relax to assist you. If you go to antenatal classes, your teacher will help you learn how to recognise when you are becoming tense and how to let go of your tension.

your head on a cupboard door, you automatically rub yourself because rubbing causes your body to make endorphins which are natural pain-killing substances. If you have a severe stomach-ache, you lie down and curl up in a ball with a hot-water bottle because warmth and being in a particular position are very comforting. Pain tells us how to help ourselves recover from injury. In labour, there is no injury taking place, but the pain teaches the woman how to give birth. She is led by it to try a variety of positions to increase her comfort and by moving around and using different positions, she also helps her baby's head press down firmly all around the cervix so that it opens up evenly. Later in labour, her changes of position cause the baby to be shifted one way and then the other, helping him to find the easiest way down through her pelvis.

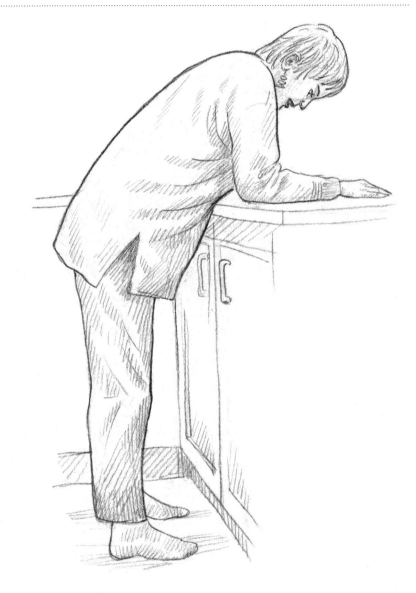

Keeping active

MOST WOMEN find that at the beginning of labour and for the first few hours, they are very restless; they have to keep on the move. This hyperactivity is a combination of being nervous and of discovering that being upright and mobile helps the pain:

'I sat down a few times, but it was uncomfortable. I just wanted to be standing up and I paced around the room.'

'I was encouraged to walk around; in fact, I was sent back up to the ward to walk around rather than staying in delivery.'

'I was in a rocking chair for most of the night. I asked for a rocking chair and it was really good.'

Nature is very rhythmical – the beating of the heart, the pattern of sleeping and waking, a woman's monthly cycle – and the way in which contractions rise up to a climax and then subside is also rhythmical. It's probably not surprising, therefore, that women often choose rhythmical activities to help them cope: *'There was only a small space in the delivery room to walk about in, so it was a sort of rhythmic pacing up and down, trying to relax and concentrate.'*

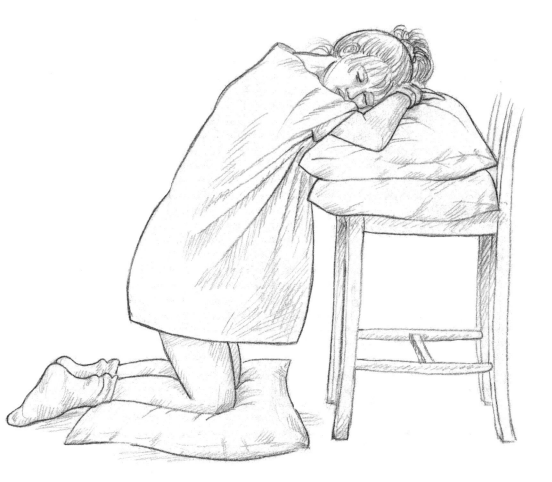

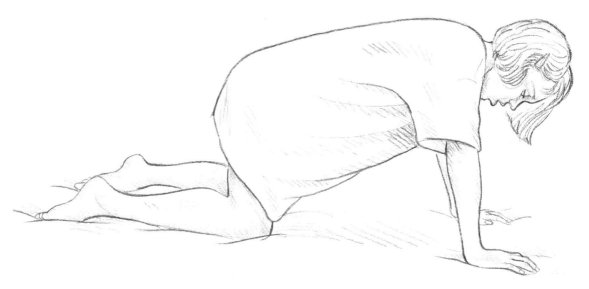

'*What made pain worse was being static at any stage. What made the pain better was leaning forwards, swaying my hips from side to side and then round and round.*'

Later on, when labour has progressed and contractions are stronger, women move around less, but they still rarely choose to sit or lie down:

'*I couldn't walk or stand up even; I just had to kneel. It was so painful.*'

'*As the contractions got a bit stronger, I went onto my hands and knees and it seemed to ease the weight on my back.*'

'*I just didn't want to lie down on the bed because it made the contractions so much more difficult to cope with.*'

Touch during labour

HAVING THE FREEDOM to move around during labour and choose the positions which make you most comfortable is immensely helpful. Equally important is the support which you receive from your labour supporter and midwife. Their words of encouragement are vital, but even more important is the way in which they touch and hold you.

Having your back rubbed or massaged during labour is helpful not only because the pressure is comforting, but also because the physical contact with someone who cares for you and is trying hard to help you is the most wonderful form of pain relief. Women need to be loved during labour!

'It was the lower spine where I was getting the pain and just pressure or rubbing it seemed to take the edge off.'

'What really helped me was the massage – I wanted more, harder, harder. It was wonderful. I suppose it added pressure but was taking it away at the same time. It was brilliant.'

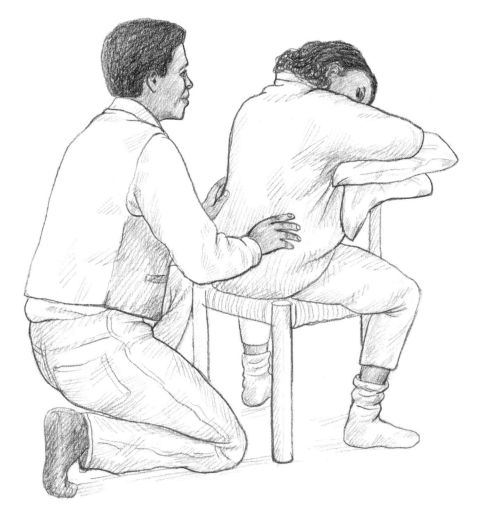

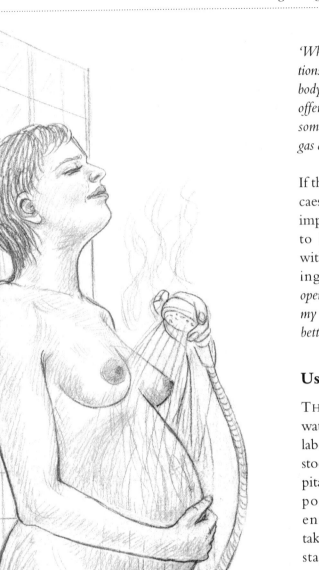

'When I was having contractions, I needed to hold somebody's hand. Gas and air was offered to me, but I grabbed somebody's hand rather than gas and air; that got me over it.'

If the baby is being born by caesarean section, it is still important for the woman to have physical contact with someone who is caring for her: 'During the operation, he was just stroking my head which made me feel better.'

Using water

THE CAPACITY of warm water to soothe the pain of labour is now well understood. More and more hospitals are installing birthing pools and midwives are encouraging women to take a bath during the first stage of labour although not all are happy for them to give birth in the water. If the mother is labouring at home, she is free to use her own bath or shower as she pleases. Some women describe how their pain almost magically disappeared once they got into the water:

'The pool looked incredibly inviting. I got in when I was 6 cms dilated. It was fantastic – everything I'd imagined. I could fully relax between contractions rather than waiting in dread for the next one. Jason rubbed the small of my back and the effect of that, along with the warm water was just wonderful.'

'I had to be in the shower. I had to have really hot water pounding down on my back.'

However, as with every other form of pain relief in labour, what suits one woman will not suit another. Each woman is unique in the way in which her body responds to pain and in the things she finds helpful. For some women, getting into a pool is definitely not soothing:

'I felt very vulnerable in the bath. It wasn't a big round bath, just a normal thin long bath and I had quite a violent contraction as I got in and I kept thinking, "I wish I could get out". I wanted to be standing up and I didn't feel very secure or very confident in the bath.'

If you are able to use a bath or birthing pool during labour, and the idea appeals to you, give it a try. If you don't find the water helpful, you can simply get out and try something else. There's nothing lost.

Breathing and relaxation

ANTENATAL CLASSES often spend a lot of time helping women understand their breathing patterns and teaching them how to use their breathing to cope with pain in labour. Relaxation is also likely to feature high on the course agenda. But can women put into practice what they have learned in their classes? Breathing techniques certainly seem to be helpful: *'What made it better for me was the breathing, the breathing exercises. They really do work. You don't think they will, but they do. You've got to concentrate; if you let your mind wander, then you've lost it. You've got to concentrate totally on the breathing you're doing.'*

'For me, it was breathing that helped with the contractions. Blowing out during the contraction – that really helped me. It helped me so much that I was 8 cms dilated when I got to the hospital.'

ALTERNATIVE FORMS OF PAIN RELIEF

Acupuncture

Aromatherapy

Homoeopathy

Hypnotherapy

Reflexology

All these can offer help with pregnancy and postnatal problems. They can also be used to help a woman cope with pain in labour. Some midwives are trained in a particular therapy and may be allowed by their hospital or health authority to offer it to the women in their care. Alternative therapists take a holistic approach to care, that is, they treat people as a whole, looking at their personality types and moods as much as at their bodily symptoms. Research into alternative therapies is still in its infancy and, at present, evidence that they are safe and effective is largely hearsay. However, more and more research is being carried out and people who practise as alternative therapists are increasingly regulated by Associations which have Codes of Professional Conduct in the same way as do orthodox health professionals.

If you are interested in using one of these therapies, you can:

● Talk to other women who have tried it
● Obtain a list of registered or trained therapists
● Contact a local therapist and ask how much he/she charges for a consultation and what kind of help you can expect to get
● Talk to your midwife about the therapy you are interested in: there may be a local health professional who has some knowledge of it or who is trained as a therapist
● Read books and magazine articles and get as much information as you can.

Alternative therapies can be used to treat morning sickness, varicose veins, haemorrhoids, headaches, heartburn and depression; they can also be used to help with slow labours, to alleviate pain in labour, and to control bleeding after labour; they can be tried for comforting babies who cry a lot, who suffer from colic or who have been traumatised by their birth.

Relaxing during labour is not easy, but women who try to relax find that it makes an appreciable difference: *'It's very difficult to relax, isn't it, because you feel your tummy go hard and the rest of you seems to clench up. You find that you are even clenching your fists, and your teeth are grinding together, and you have to force yourself to relax and calm down. It does help when you relax, it definitely does.'*

'I tried to relax during the contractions and I took my walkman and we'd taped my favourite songs and I listened to them over and over again and that helped me relax.'

You will almost certainly
find that not all of what
you have learnt in ante-
natal classes or from reading books or from
listening to other women
is helpful on the day. It's
perhaps best to think of
the breathing techniques
and the positions and the
relaxation exercises
which you practise as
tools for labour. When
the day comes, you look
through the tools you
have prepared and
choose the ones you
want. The rest you put
by, perhaps to be used
later, or perhaps not at
all:

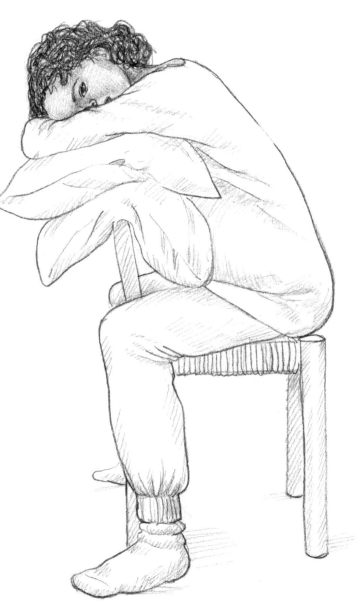

*'Labour felt just like a very
strong period pain and being
touched made it worse. All
the massage we practised –
I didn't want to be touched
at all. Using different positions, though, felt completely
natural.'*

*'My breathing went com-
pletely out of the window. To begin with, I felt I was doing the right thing,
but the nurses said I wasn't. I was panting when I wasn't supposed to be and
I think it was panic and I just forgot everything we'd talked about except
making a noise. Shouting was brilliant!'*

MEDICAL FORMS OF PAIN RELIEF

IF YOU are having a home birth, you can use gas and air (which the midwife may call Entonox) to help you or you could have pethidine although this is unusual. You can also use a TENS machine. In hospital, you can use all these and you could also have an epidural. What you have to decide is whether the amount of help you will get from using drugs in labour is sufficient to outweigh the disadvantages of having them.

Entonox

LOTS OF women find Entonox (or 'gas and air') helpful:

'I have a friend who has just had a baby boy, a big baby. She is five foot; she had a forty hours' labour and managed with gas and air.'

'I thought gas and air was wonderful. I wanted to take it home with me!'

'Breathing the gas and air helped me control my breathing.'

'I wanted to push and the midwife kept telling me not to push because I wasn't fully dilated; that was the worst point. That's when I started on the gas and air and it really helped.'

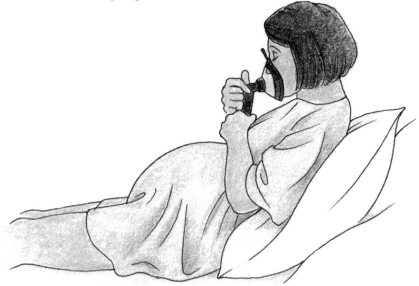

METHODS OF PAIN RELIEF

Entonox

The Facts:

- It's made up of 50% oxygen and 50% nitrous oxide
- You take the gas in either through a rubber mask which goes over your face or through a mouth piece which you put between your lips and which you can grasp with your teeth. You breathe in and out through the mouthpiece or mask
- The trick is to begin breathing the gas deeply and evenly as soon as you feel a contraction coming. Don't wait until the contraction reaches its peak and is very painful. If you start taking the gas when the contraction starts, it will build up gradually in your blood stream so that by the time the contraction is at its height, you will be getting maximum pain relief
- You must hold the mouthpiece or mask yourself – when you have had enough, you will start to feel slightly light-headed, your muscles will relax and your hand will drop away from your face. If someone holds the mask for you, you run the risk of taking too much gas.

The Advantages:

- You are in control of Entonox – you use it as and when you want
- Its effects are short-lived; in between contractions, the light-headedness will disappear
- Entonox has no known harmful effects on your baby; in fact, the oxygen part is probably good for him.

The Disadvantages:

- Entonox is only a mild pain-killer; it can take the edge off contractions but it won't take the pain away entirely
- If you use it for a long time, you may find that your mouth becomes very dry. Your labour supporter needs to give you sips of water to drink in between each contraction
- Some women say that Entonox makes them feel sick; in fact, the sickness is probably due to the rubber face mask rather than the gas and you should always ask for a mouthpiece if you don't like the mask.

But it doesn't suit everybody: *'As a neurotic dental patient, I have been brought up on gas and air. I was disappointed that the Entonox mixture at the hospital was a weaker variety than the one I was used to. Also I didn't like having the mask over my mouth and nose. Instead of being able to concentrate on going into myself, I found the Entonox an unnecessary distraction and it also made me feel sick.'*

Some women find that gas and air is not enough to help them through the most difficult part of their labour and want to choose a stronger form of pain relief. You can try the gas and air to see how helpful it is and if you don't like it, you can simply put it aside and try something else. The same applies to TENS.

METHODS OF PAIN RELIEF

TENS

(Transcutaneous Electrical Nerve Stimulation) Two pairs of self-adhesive electrodes are put on your back, one on either side of your spine. These are connected by wires to a small box with a dial or dials, and a boost button control. The dials control the strength and frequency of the pulses of electricity which the machine gives out. These pulses block the pain messages being sent to the brain by your uterus and cervix and also stimulate your body to release natural pain-killing substances called endorphins. Research suggests that TENS is most effective for pain relief if you try it out during the last weeks of your pregnancy and then use it from the start of labour and gradually adjust the level of the machine's output to match the increasing strength of contractions. The boost button allows you to obtain maximum output from the machine at the height of difficult contractions.

- You control the TENS machine and if you don't like it, you can take it off

- Women who are having their second or subsequent baby often report finding TENS very helpful; first-time mothers may need to supplement it with other forms of pain relief

- There's no reason to believe that TENS does any harm to the baby, but there's no long-term research to prove it is harmless.

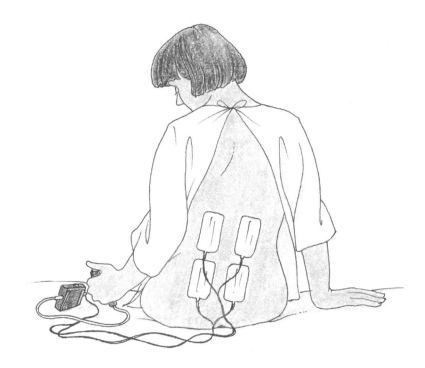

TENS

TENS HAS BEEN used by physiotherapists to treat muscle injuries and chronic back pain for many years, but it's only been used in childbirth relatively recently. It seems to work most effectively when the woman starts using the machine at the very beginning of her labour. Although, like gas and air, it's not a very strong form of pain relief, some women find it helpful, especially in early labour:

'I put the TENS machine on soon after I arrived at the hospital and I found it really useful and I got to 6 cms with just the TENS which was good.'

'I tried the TENS unit because I'd decided that I didn't want pethidine or gas and air. It sends little shivers, like pins and needles, down your back and I thought it was good and I would have it again. I don't think it did actually take the pain away, but it takes your mind off it.'

Others are less convinced of its benefits: *'The contractions came so quickly, it didn't have time to work.'*

Pethidine

PETHIDINE IS still widely used for pain relief in labour, although not nearly as much as it was before epidurals came on the scene. Meptid and diamorphine have threatened at various times to take its place, but this has not happened. Yet pethidine rarely gets rave reviews from women who have used it. Some women appreciate it because it helps them to have a rest, perhaps even a few hours sleep during labour, but others find that the drowsiness which pethidine causes is insufficient to carry them over the top of contractions and makes them feel completely out of control of what is happening to them.

'I found the pethidine didn't help because I woke at the height of each contraction and wasn't able to cope with the pain at that point.'

'I was tired, exhausted; they said, "You need pethidine." Why do they offer pethidine when you are losing control? It makes you lose control more.'

METHODS OF PAIN RELIEF

Pethidine

The Facts:
- Pethidine is a drug which is related to morphine. It tends to make you drowsy and possibly disorientated
- It is given by injection, generally into your thigh or bottom
- A standard dose is 100mgs, but it is possible to give less. A smaller dose is appropriate if you are small or lightly built. Pethidine can be given more than once during labour
- The midwife will not want you to have pethidine if she thinks you are within a few hours of giving birth. This is because pethidine crosses the placenta and will affect your baby most strongly if it has been given shortly before you deliver.

The Advantages:
- If a woman is extremely tense during her labour, contractions may become chaotic and not very good at opening up the cervix. Pethidine is useful for helping a woman relax so that her uterus finds its rhythm again
- Some women will tell you that pethidine was marvellous for them because it allowed them to have a much-needed rest during labour and helped them cope with the pain of contractions.

The Disadvantages:
- Pethidine not only acts to relieve pain, but also affects your breathing which becomes shallower and slower. Because it crosses the placenta, it may also affect the baby's breathing after he is born
- Some women say that pethidine made them so drowsy that they were not even aware that their baby was being born. Missing the birth in this way can cause a woman to be very unhappy about her labour afterwards

- Some women find that pethidine makes them unaware of the gradual build-up of a contraction, but is not strong enough to carry them over its peak. The result is that they tend to 'wake up' at the most painful moment of each contraction
- Pethidine can make mothers feel very sick and for this reason, it is often given with another drug to help control sickness.

Diamorphine (heroin)

The Facts:
- This is a drug which is very similar to pethidine but it is used much less frequently.

The Advantages:
- Some health professionals feel that it is a better pain-killer than pethidine
- Women who have used it describe a pleasant feeling of detachment from their labours.

The Disadvantages:
- Diamorphine, like pethidine, passes through the placenta to the baby and may be more likely to affect the baby's breathing than pethidine.

Meptid

The Facts:
- This is another alternative to pethidine. It may not be available at the hospital where you have booked.

The Advantages:
- There is some research to suggest that meptid has less effect on the baby's breathing than pethidine.

The Disadvantages:
- The side-effects for the mother are similar to those of pethidine and may be worse in terms of causing sickness.

Pethidine is least satisfactory when the woman is so completely knocked out by it that she's not even aware her baby has been born: *'Labour is just a blur to me; I couldn't tell you how Sophie was born.'*

Where epidurals are praised for helping the woman feel is control of her labour, some women will not consider having pethidine because they fear it might deprive them of the first moments of their babies' lives: *'The only thing I've got quite clear is that I want to be conscious, I want to be there. Anything that's likely to cloud your mind like pethidine, I would not want because it's very important to be completely alert when you meet your baby.'*

If you do decide to have pethidine in labour because you want something stronger than gas and air but don't want an epidural, discuss with your midwife whether having 25mg or 50mg instead of the standard 100mg might be a good idea. Remember that you can always have more pethidine if you need it, but once it's been given, you can't have it taken away if it turns out to have been too much.

Epidurals

IT IS ALWAYS possible to find a lot of women who are strongly in favour of epidurals because they feel that an epidural allows a woman to regain control of her labour and of her dignity: *'I remember seeing this woman in labour on a video who'd had an epidural and she was telling jokes. She was screaming beforehand.'*

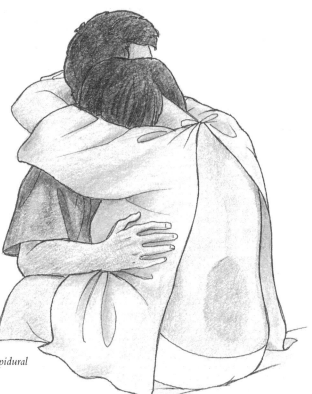

Getting into position for an epidural

METHODS OF PAIN RELIEF

Epidurals

The Facts:

- An epidural is set up by an anaesthetist; if the hospital is busy, you may have to wait until an anaesthetist is available. You can't have an epidural for a home birth!

- The procedure is as follows: first a doctor puts a drip into your arm. This is because an epidural may cause your blood pressure to drop suddenly and the drip means that fluids can be given straight into your blood stream to bring your blood pressure back up again. Next the anaesthetist sprays the bottom of your back with a cold solution to numb the skin. He or she then puts a hollow needle into your back, feeling carefully for the right spot just outside the protective layers which surround the spinal cord. A narrow tube called a catheter is threaded through the needle and the needle is taken out of your back. The catheter is taped over your shoulder and the anaesthetist injects a pain-killing solution into the top end. You may feel a cold sensation in your back soon afterwards and be asked to lie first on one side then on the other to help the solution spread evenly. Within a few seconds, you start to lose the feeling in your legs and the contractions disappear. The epidural can be 'topped up' by the midwife when you start to feel the contractions again

- If you have an epidural during the early part of labour, you may have a tube or (catheter) put into your bladder so that urine can drain freely into a bag attached to the tube. This is necessary because you cannot tell when you need to go to the toilet and a full bladder will make it more difficult for the baby to be born.

The Advantages:

- Epidurals give many women complete relief from labour pain
- They can help a mother feel 'in control' of her labour again when she had previously felt out of control because of the intensity of her contractions
- If the mother needs stitches after giving birth, an epidural will provide pain relief while the stitching is carried out
- If a caesarean section becomes necessary during labour, the epidural can be used as an anaesthetic for the operation rather than the mother needing to have a general anaesthetic. This means that she can be awake when her baby is born.

The Disadvantages:

- A significant proportion of women, perhaps as many as 10–15%, do not get complete pain relief from an epidural. Some find that they are numb down one side of the lower part of their body, but not the other. Some women describe 'windows of pain' when a small patch on their tummy or back seems not to have been affected by the epidural and they feel their contractions intensely in this one spot
- An epidural may make some women feel very *out* of control of their labour. Because they have a tube in their back, a drip in their arm and perhaps a catheter in their bladder, and have no sensation of contractions at all, they feel entirely dependent on health professionals to deliver their baby and totally uninvolved in the birth themselves
- If the epidural is still working in the second stage of labour when the baby is being born, the mother may not be able to push effectively and so runs a higher risk of needing to have her baby delivered by forceps or suction

METHODS OF PAIN RELIEF

- Sometimes the epidural needle pierces the covering surrounding the spinal cord and this means that the fluid which bathes the spinal cord leaks out slightly. The mother finds that she has an overpowering headache after the labour which makes her quite unable to look after her baby. It may then be necessary for a doctor to take some blood from her and inject it into her back to seal the hole made by the epidural needle

- There is some research to suggest that a number of women may suffer from chronic low backache, shoulder ache and tingling of their arms and legs for weeks, months or even years after having an epidural. It is not certain whether these effects are due to the epidural itself or to the fact that the mother tends to remain in one position for the duration of her labour.

An epidural can transform a labour which is frightening to the woman because of the amount of pain involved or which threatens to be very long and difficult into an experience which she remembers with pleasure and satisfaction: *'We were sitting there for two hours and I only got to 1 cm. And I was really relieved when they said, "Have an epidural" and I went to sleep for two hours and when I woke, I was 10 cms. And that's the way to do it! It was brilliant. No suffering or pain at all.'*

'I was given a drip and had an epidural which I thought was very good. I was very with it when the baby was born and it was a positive experience and I wouldn't rule out having an epidural again.'

'You don't know how you're going to react. I found the labour incredibly hard. The epidural made it OK for me. I was so glad to have it.'

However, although epidurals are now replacing pethidine as the principal form of pain relief for labouring women, especially those having their first babies, they may not take away all the pain of the contractions. A few women find that their epidural is only partly effective: *'I found the epidural quite frightening. It didn't work as high up as it should and I could still feel the contractions pushing up into my ribs and it was most peculiar.'*

METHODS OF PAIN RELIEF

Spinals

The Facts:
A spinal anaesthetic is an injection given into the lower part of the mother's back. It can only be given once so the pain relief is short term.

The Advantages:
● A spinal anaesthetic can be given more quickly than an epidural and its effect is almost immediate. It is therefore very useful when the mother needs some speedy pain relief to help her such as when, for example, her baby needs to be born with the help of forceps or suction
● A spinal can be used for a caesarean section provided that the obstetrician is sure the operation will be uncomplicated. A spinal wears off much more quickly than an epidural so the mother soon has normal sensation again.

The Disadvantages:
● There is a greater risk of a sudden fall in the mother's blood pressure with a spinal than with an epidural
● The injection pierces the covering around the spinal cord so that fluid may leak out causing the mother to have a severe headache after the birth of her baby
● A spinal offers only short-term pain relief and so is no use if the labour is expected to be long.

Because an anaesthetist must be called to set up an epidural and he or she may bring another doctor to assist in the procedure, the delivery room may suddenly fill up with people. Some women greatly dislike the loss of privacy which an epidural entails: *'What I didn't like was that I had to lie on the bed all the time and there were a lot of doctors around and I would rather just have had my husband and a midwife.'*

It may be several hours after the birth of her baby before a woman who has had an epidural completely regains the normal sensations in her legs and lower body and there can also be longer-term side-effects to cope with. There is research now to suggest that epidurals may be responsible for some chronic back problems: *'I've had a lot of backache since I gave birth to Paul and I'm not sure if it's because his head was in a funny position or whether it's due to the epidural.'*

PREPARING TO COPE WITH PAIN

WHILE YOU are pregnant, you can think about how you're going to cope with pain in labour and which methods of pain relief, whether natural or medical, you would prefer to use. Some women make a firm decision about pain relief before labour starts and stick to it: *'I was quite adamant beforehand that I wasn't going to use any pain relief because I hate things like needles and I wanted to be fully aware of what was going on and I just felt I could manage without any drugs. And I wanted to show my boyfriend as well because he thinks I'm a real wimp! In the end, just the massage got me through.'*

But other women find that keeping an open mind might have been better: *'I had written all across my notes: "Does not want an epidural". Did I feel a fool! When I arrived, I was screaming for one. I was most abusive to my husband who was reminding me that I didn't want to have an epidural. So I think the important thing is to go in open-minded.'*

It is probably not wise to have made all your decisions about which forms of pain relief to use in labour before the day arrives. It is helpful, however, to find out beforehand about what your options are if you are having a home birth, and which forms of pain relief are most commonly used at the local maternity units if you are going to have your baby in hospital. If you are almost certain that you will want an epidural, you need to choose a hospital where epidurals are available twenty-four hours a day. If you feel that you want to avoid having a lot of drugs in labour, you might decide to have a home birth or to go to a hospital which has a reputation for helping women cope without drugs. You could also talk to your labour supporter about your preferences for pain relief. Being prepared is more than half the battle: *'You know that you can't imagine the pain beforehand, but if you prepare yourself by getting lots of information and you know what your choices are, you're giving yourself the best chance. Before I knew anything, I was so anxious, but now I feel I am armed and that I have something to hold on to.'*

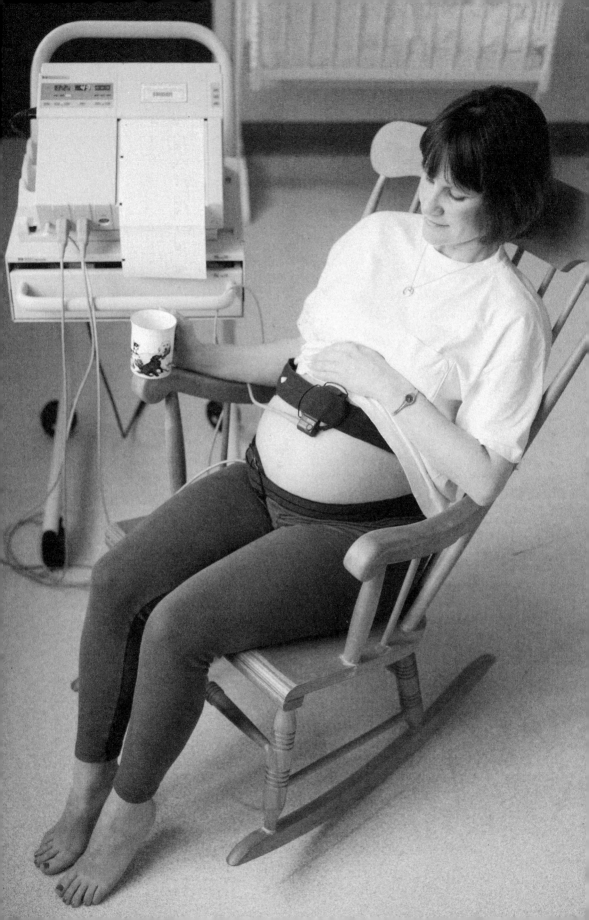

CHAPTER *six* *Interventions in labour*

PREGNANCY AND LABOUR are not illnesses. Having a baby is a normal part of a woman's life. The vast majority of women are perfectly able to give birth to their babies with no assistance at all. This is probably especially true of women in the highly developed parts of the world who have been privileged to have a good diet from birth, and who have grown into healthy young women. In this country, where organised health care has been available for fifty years, today's childbearing women are the daughters of women who were themselves fit and well nourished and they are probably the grand daughters of women who were also very healthy. After generations of good health, the risks of childbearing become ever smaller. The evidence for this can be seen in the statistics for the number of women and babies who die around childbirth. Nowadays, hardly anyone knows of a woman who died whilst having a baby; mercifully few women have suffered the overwhelming grief of giving birth to a stillborn baby.

So having a baby in the UK today is very safe because we are, by and large, a healthy nation. We are able to drink clean water; the sewerage system is efficient; most of us are well housed so that we don't suffer from the health problems associated with living in damp or insanitary conditions. It is mainly because of improvements in people's living conditions over the last century that childbearing has become so safe. The part played by modern obstetrics is far less significant.

This is not to say that no one benefits from the fact that doctors and hospitals are now heavily involved in childbirth. For a small proportion of women, the availability of such things as ultrasound monitoring, drugs to induce labour, forceps and ventouse to help babies be born, and caesarean sections makes childbearing safe for them when it wouldn't have been otherwise. For these women, the technology of birth can literally be life-saving.

UNDERSTANDING YOUR CARE IN LABOUR

Before you agree to have any medical procedure or intervention in labour, make sure that you understand exactly why your midwife or doctor is suggesting it and what it involves. Your mind will be much more at rest during your labour and you will feel far happier afterwards if you have had all your questions answered.

The Questions to Ask

- What are the benefits for me and my baby if I have this procedure?

- Are there any risks?

- What exactly does the procedure involve?

- If I agree to it, is it likely that I will need to have other interventions during my labour?

- Is there anything else that could be tried before doing this?

- What might happen if I decided to wait a little before making up my mind?

- What might happen if I decide not to go ahead with this procedure?

In the past, however, the technology tended to get out of hand and procedures which were useful for a small number of women were applied to every woman. Induction rates in the 1970s climbed to as many as 60% of births in some hospitals; women were being induced not because their babies were at risk but because it was more convenient if they gave birth at certain times of the day or on certain days of the week. This was clearly a crazy state of affairs. It has to be recognised that every intervention in the natural process of giving birth will carry a certain amount of risk with it. The more frequently interventions are used for women who don't need them, the more likely it is that, overall, their drawbacks will outweigh their benefits.

Over the last few years, women's organisations and health professionals have joined together to question some of the interventions which are routinely used in childbirth. Important books have been written which show, for example, that for most women it is no safer to have a baby in hospital than at home; that electronic monitoring is no better at detecting babies who are responding badly to labour than less intrusive forms of monitoring such as Sonicaid and the midwife's ear-trumpet; that breaking the bag of waters around the baby in order to speed up labour is only likely to reduce the length of labour by about half an hour. As more and more research has shown how safe birth is and how harmful it can be to interfere with the natural process, there has been a swing away from interfering with labour. Midwives in particular are now generally keen to protect the woman in labour from unnecessary interventions and to encourage her to trust her own body and to cope on her own. More and more women are recognising that they have considerable personal resources for coping with labour and that they do not need to behave like patients, lying on a hospital bed while they are giving birth. Instead, they can act as independent, healthy adults, choosing to do what makes them most comfortable, being upright and mobile in labour and delivering their babies kneeling, or squatting or on all fours.

There is also a greater understanding nowadays of the important part which emotions play in the process of having a baby. If the mother is frightened and tense, these feelings may affect her labour and make it slower and more difficult. She is likely to have a far easier time if she is well supported, kept informed about how her labour is going and consulted about the care she is being offered.

INTERVENTIONS IN LABOUR

- Induction of labour – Having your labour started off artificially

- Vaginal examination – (VE) – Having an internal when the midwife puts her fingers into the vagina to see how far open the cervix is and what position the baby is lying in

- Artificial rupture of membranes – (ARM) – Having the bag of waters broken

- Acceleration of labour – Having a drip to make contractions stronger

- Abdominal monitoring or fetal scalp electrode monitoring – Being monitored electronically either by having two transducers strapped onto your abdomen or by having an electrode clipped onto the baby's head

- Assisted delivery with forceps or ventouse – Having forceps or suction to help the baby be born

- Caesarean section (may be abbreviated to ECS – elective caesarean section, or LSCS – lower segment caesarean section).

Magazines about birth and parenting are urging women to make their own decisions about what happens in labour based on their personal preferences and the information which they get from health professionals. Women now have the opportunity to take responsibility for the birth of their babies; this is both rewarding and frightening. However, parenthood is all about making decisions for our children, and it seems logical that we should start making those decisions when our babies are still in the uterus or while they are being born.

When women take responsibility alongside health professionals for making decisions about their labour, what they might once have seen as an unwanted intervention becomes something they have chosen to have:

'An intervention is something that's done to you without your consent. If I want to have a caesarean section, that's not an intervention; or if I want to have an epidural, that's not an intervention. To me an intervention means things being taken out of your control or something that you're pressurised into having.'

'Even if you have interventions, you can still have an element of control if you've discussed them.'

Women are quite wise enough to know that sometimes interventions are very necessary, and they are not going to make decisions which put either themselves or their babies at risk: *'I don't see forceps and stitches − all those sorts of things − as interventions if they're necessary. I'll accept them if they're needed and I won't see them as interventions but as part of the process of helping the baby out safely.'*

'I would want as natural a delivery as possible, but if the baby's in distress and I understand why they are recommending something, I'll go along with what they say and I'll be quite happy with that.'

THE MOTHER is the person with the greatest interest in her baby's well-being, and the decisions she takes will reflect this concern that no harm should come to her child. Few women will choose to go against what health professionals recommend provided that they are given reasons for the advice they are being offered. And most women will feel far happier about their care if they have been consulted about it.

INDUCTION − GETTING INFORMATION

ALTHOUGH WOMEN used regularly to be induced when they were exactly forty weeks pregnant or just a few days over their due date, attitudes towards induction have changed and most medical and mid-wifery staff now consider it quite safe for a woman to go at least two weeks late. There are all sorts of ways of finding out whether the baby is still doing well in the womb, and if he is, there seems little reason to disturb him. The vast majority of women will have delivered their babies by 42 weeks of pregnancy and nearly all of them by 43 weeks.

However, it's still true to say that obstetricians have different views about when a woman's labour should be induced: *'The midwife told me that one of the obstetricians here is keen on inducing when you're a week over, more so than the others.'*

The very fact that there are differences of opinion suggests that the decision about induction is often not a clear-cut one, and so there is no reason why *your* opinion shouldn't be taken into account. You may have very strong feelings one way or the other about the merits of a prolonged pregnancy: *'I think if the baby's not ready to come out, it's for a reason. They come when they want to come and we should leave well alone unless the baby's not doing well.'*

On the other hand, it can seem an interminably long wait for some women: *'My doctor said that he is happy to let his ladies go over by three weeks. I feel like tearing my hair out!'*

Some women are surprised to find that they have a choice about whether to be induced: *'At my hospital, they leave you 10 days late and then they induce you. I didn't realise you had any other option.'*

Of course, there are some circumstances in which the health professionals and the mother are likely to feel that there is no choice and that an induction is very necessary because both the mother and the baby will be better off if the baby is born. One of these circumstances is when the woman has very high blood pressure: *'Throughout my pregnancy, I had high blood pressure and I knew there was a danger to both myself and the baby. So I was happy to be induced.'*

Getting information about the induction sometimes depends on having the courage to ask questions: *'After we started asking questions, they offered us an alternative, but they didn't offer us that until we started asking questions. In the end, we didn't go for the induction. I went thirteen days over.'*

REASONS WHY LABOUR MIGHT BE INDUCED

1. *The mother has gone over her due date by more than two weeks.* Induction used to be offered when the mother was just a few days past her due date, but in the majority of cases, it is now considered to be quite safe to wait until 42 weeks.

2. *Pre-eclampsia*: the mother's blood pressure is very high and she has protein in her urine.

3. *The baby seems to have stopped growing* and the mother is feeling fewer movements than she did.

4. *The mother's waters have broken but contractions have not started.* Induction may be suggested because of the risk of the mother's uterus or the baby becoming infected from the bacteria in the vagina.

5. There are a number of other less common reasons for an induction:

- The mother has previously given birth to a very large baby and the doctors want to prevent this baby growing as large
- The mother has previously had a very fast labour and she wants to be sure that this labour takes place in a safe environment
- The mother has genital herpes or warts and the baby needs to be born at a time when the warts are not 'active' or weepy
- The mother's baby has died in utero and she doesn't want to wait for labour to start naturally.

Not being given a reason for the induction is entirely unsatisfactory to most women and some will demand to be told: *'When induction was first mentioned, he just said: "Come in tomorrow", and walked out of the room. I said, "Excuse me!" It was a trainee doctor and as soon as I started to ask questions, he said, "I'll have to go and get the consultant." The consultant came and was a bit defensive to start with because we were saying things like, "What will happen if we don't have the induction? Is there any alternative? What other choices have we got?" – in other words, asking for the sort of information we needed to make a decision. And eventually I said to him, "Please just give us all the information you can and then could you let us have a few minutes to think about things on our own." Once I had calmed down, he did too, and he did give us the information and we talked about it and he came back five minutes later and we told him our decision. He was quite reasonable about what we wanted and there was no shouting at all!'*

Very often, a calm but assertive approach is successful in getting the information you need and establishing a relationship of mutual trust and respect with your professional carers.

Alternatives to medical induction

THERE ARE ways of inducing labour which you can try for yourself if you are well over your dates and don't want to be induced. These are neatly summarised in the words of one woman: *'Hot curry, hot bath, hot sex!'*

While there is no research evidence to bear out the effectiveness of the first two, the last certainly has its roots in physiology. The semen which the man ejaculates during love-making contains substances called prostaglandins. Prostaglandin pessaries are often used to induce labour.

What does induction feel like?

YOU MIGHT be asked to come into hospital the evening before your induction, or you might already be in hospital because you haven't been well. The night spent anticipating labour can be a very long one: *'When Steve went home, I felt very, very small, especially in the dark with everyone else asleep. I was awake all night and I wanted to go home.'*

It is not uncommon for induced labours to be fast and furious. Women can find that rather than having time to adjust to a labour which builds up gradually, they are plunged immediately into very strong and frequent contractions: *'I was induced and the effect of the pessaries was nothing one minute – no labour at all – and then suddenly contractions lasting one minute or a minute and a half with thirty seconds off in between. I had been examined shortly before they started me off and I wasn't dilated at all, and in about three hours, I went to 8 cms. Psychologically, I had no idea what was going on, so for me it was a lot more traumatic than I thought it would be.'*

HOW IS LABOUR INDUCED?

There are three methods:

● Prostaglandin pessaries: pessaries are oval tablets of jelly which the midwife puts into the woman's vagina close to the cervix. Pessaries are good for 'ripening' the cervix: that is, they help make the cervix soft and ready for labour. After the midwife has given the pessaries, the mother is monitored in bed for an hour or so with two transducers strapped to her abdomen to see whether contractions are beginning and how her baby is reacting to them. (Prostaglandin can also be given in the form of gel.)

● Breaking the waters: if the mother's cervix has opened a little, the midwife can use an amnihook which looks like a very long crotchet hook to break the bag of waters around the baby. The mother lies on her back at the end of the bed with her knees drawn up and apart and covered in green, sterile towels. The waters drain into a bucket placed underneath the bed.

● A syntocinon drip: the mother is given a drip which contains syntocinon, an artificial form of oxytocin, the hormone which makes the uterus contract. The amount of syntocinon given to the mother is gradually increased to mimic the build-up of oxytocin in a normal labour.

PRE-ECLAMPSIA (PREGNANCY INDUCED HYPERTENSION PIH)

● What is it?
  A disease of pregnancy.

● What signs and symptoms are there?
  ● Protein in the urine
  ● High blood pressure
  ● Headaches and spots before the eyes
  ● Sickness
  ● Pain in the top half of the abdomen.
Although each of these last three symptoms could be due to something other than pre-eclampsia, you should certainly contact your midwife or doctor at once if you have any of them, as they might indicate very serious pre-eclampsia requiring urgent medical attention.

● How do I know if I've got it?
  Each time your midwife comes to check you at home during your pregnancy, or you go for an antenatal appointment at your doctor's surgery or at the hospital, your urine will be tested to see if there is any protein in it. The midwife will also take your blood pressure. These tests are designed to help your health carers find out if you have pre-eclampsia or are at risk of developing it.

● What are the problems for me and my baby if I have pre-eclampsia?
  If your blood pressure is high, the placenta doesn't work well and your baby may not get all the food and oxygen he needs to grow properly. Very high blood pressure is also bad for you as it can damage your kidneys and may cause you to have fits (although this is extremely rare).

● What will happen if I get pre-eclampsia?
  Your doctor or midwife may want to see you more regularly to check your blood pressure and test your urine. You may be told to rest at home or asked to come into hospital to rest, although there's no proof that resting helps pre-eclampsia. If your pre-eclampsia is very bad, you will be offered an induction to start you off in labour, or a caesarean section so that your baby can be born before either of you comes to any harm.

The opposite case is when the woman has an induction and nothing happens: *'I had the pessaries and Mel went home. I wasn't worried; I was just bored; there was nothing happening.'*

IT MAY be necessary to give the woman pessaries on two or three occasions in order to start labour off, or to try several different methods of induction before contractions begin.

Even with good support, women often need more help from drugs to cope with the pain of an induced labour than they would otherwise have done:

'*If I was induced again, I would certainly have another epidural because I couldn't cope without one.*'

'*The pessaries didn't work, so they set up a drip and I felt I'd just gone bang – right into it. I straight away wanted an epidural.*'

Induced labours also have a greater chance of ending in emergency caesareans than normal labours. Sometimes an induction leads to another intervention and then to another, a phenomenon which has been described as 'the cascade of intervention': '*I had the pessaries and then they broke my waters because they said it might speed labour up which it didn't; it didn't do anything at all. Then I was all hooked up to the monitors. I was in so much pain, I had to have the epidural and by this time, understandably, the baby had a bit of distress so they took the decision, because I wasn't dilating, to do a caesarean.*'

Fortunately, not all women have such an unsatisfactory experience and many are pleased that the long days of waiting after their due date has passed are coming to an end: '*They gave me the prostaglandin gel on Sunday evening and said that nothing would happen overnight and it didn't except for some backache. Then they gave me more at eight in the morning and monitored me for half an hour. I put my TENS machine on at ten, and the contractions just started getting stronger and stronger and I went into full labour which I thought was going to last for hours and hours, but she was born at twenty to eleven, so it was wonderful. I would be induced again if I was late; there are pros and cons. I was very lucky that it all went very quickly and I only had to have gel.*'

OTHER METHODS OF INTERVENTION

Speeding labour up

IN SOME hospitals, it is very common for women to have their waters broken during labour. The reason often given for this is that it will speed labour up. Or a drip containing artificial oxytocin may be started in order to make the woman's contractions stronger and her cervix open up faster. When you talk to women who have given birth, it can be surprising to discover just how many have had these kinds of

ACTIVE MANAGEMENT OF LABOUR

What is it?

In Ireland in the 1960s, a now famous obstetrician called Kieran O'Driscoll noticed that the longer a labour lasted, the more likely it was that problems would arise. He therefore set out to develop a way of managing labour which would ensure that every woman coming to his hospital delivered her baby in twelve hours or less. He used a graph to chart how quickly the mother's cervix was opening and if it was opening very slowly, her labour was speeded up either by breaking the waters around the baby or by giving her a syntocinon drip to strengthen contractions. Because the progress of labour needed to be observed very carefully, a midwife was assigned to each woman to be with her throughout her labour until her baby was born.

Many hospitals throughout the world have taken up O'Driscoll's ideas. Check to see if your hospital follows the Active Management of Labour practices. Active Management has advantages, but also many disadvantages.

Advantages:
● Some women are relieved to know that they will not be allowed to labour for longer than a prearranged length of time. They are happy to accept a caesarean section or forceps delivery if labour continues longer than agreed

● The support offered by a midwife who stays with the mother *throughout her labour* is tremendous. A special relationship often develops which helps the mother to cope well with a labour which has been made artificially stronger or faster.

Disadvantages:
● Shorter labours are not necessarily easier to cope with than longer ones. Provided the mother can relax and is well supported, she will often cope well with a labour which is slow and builds up gradually, allowing her time to accustom herself to the increasing strength of contractions

● Not all women (or health professionals) are happy with the idea of interfering in a perfectly normal labour simply to make it faster

● Speeding the labour up artificially may mean that the mother needs to use far more pain-relieving drugs than she would have done otherwise

● Because the Active Management of Labour often involves the mother having a drip in her arm and being continuously monitored, her ability to move around is restricted and this may make labour more painful and difficult.

intervention. You may feel that nature is unlikely to require assistance on so large a scale, but it can be very difficult to challenge the system when you are not sure whether, in your case, the intervention might be justified and useful for you and your baby:

'*Of ten women I knew, all having babies at the same time, nine of them ended up having a drip to speed up labour. Now I don't believe that was necessary. But one out of ten might be necessary, and how do you know you are not that one?*'

IT'S ALWAYS a good idea to ask if you're uncertain about why a certain course of action is being suggested. Your peace of mind both during labour and afterwards will be so much greater if you understand the reasons for interventions. Health professionals are busy people and sometimes don't remember that what to them is routine is very definitely not so to you. You will nearly always find that if you ask questions, answers will be given to you: *'When I asked about things, like "What's in the drip?" because I was worried about side effects, they were very good and they did tell me. But they didn't volunteer anything; you always need to ask.'*

Having discussed the situation with your midwife and agreed together that it could be helpful for you to have your waters broken, you are much more likely to be happy with the outcome: *'They broke my waters and that was the best thing the midwife could have done. My cervix had been stuck at 3cms and afterwards, it suddenly went to 7cms. The midwife did it for a specific reason which we'd discussed and I'd agreed to.'*

When you're making your decision, however, it's important to bear in mind

SPEEDING LABOUR UP

Your midwife may suggest breaking the waters around the baby to speed labour up. This is called 'acceleration of labour'. The midwife may also want to break the waters in order to see what colour they are. If they are discoloured, this could indicate that your baby is not coping well with labour.

Here are some of the points you might want to take into consideration:

● The bag of waters is designed to act as a buffer zone around your baby, protecting him from the strength of the contractions. Once this buffer zone has been taken away, your baby may find labour much more stressful

● Research has found that breaking the waters only makes labour about half an hour shorter than it would otherwise have been

● Some women find contractions much tougher for a while after the waters are broken. Kneeling down with your shoulders lower than your bottom can help for the first contraction or two.

that, as with all other interventions, having your waters broken could in itself cause problems, or indeed, prove impossible to carry out: *'I think they tried to break the waters too soon and that's why they couldn't. Later they did and I am sure that it was because of having my waters broken that I got a uterus infection. The doctor who did it had a heavy cold. It meant I went home on antibiotics and I went back three weeks later to have more intravenous antibiotics.'*

MONITORING IN LABOUR

What does monitoring mean?

It is sometimes easy to forget that labour is an experience the baby has to go through as well as the mother. Just as the mother may sometimes find her labour hard to cope with, so may her baby. When the midwife listens to your baby's heartbeat with an ear-trumpet or Sonicaid or looks at the pattern of his heartbeat on a read-out from a monitoring machine, she is trying to understand how your baby is being affected by contractions. When your uterus contracts, your baby's umbilical cord is squeezed and his oxygen supply is reduced. His heartbeat changes when there is less oxygen. Most babies cope well with contractions and their heartbeat returns quickly to normal after each contraction has ended; a few find labour very difficult and their heartbeat becomes weaker. If it seems to the midwife and doctor that your baby's heartbeat is very slow during contractions or takes a long time to return to a normal rate in between contractions, they may want to discuss with you whether a caesarean section would be the safest way for your baby to be born.

MONITORING IN LABOUR

Statement by the Royal College of Obstetricians and Gynaecologists

New guidelines issued in 1994 by the Royal College of Obstetricians and Gynaecologists state that for women who have had normal pregnancies and who are having straightforward labours, the drawbacks of electronic monitoring outweigh the benefits. When there is no reason to fear complications, the College recommends that the best way to monitor a baby's heartbeat in labour is by listening to it every quarter of an hour with a Sonicaid or ear-trumpet.

Monitoring

BECAUSE WE live in a technological age and are increasingly used to relying on technology at home and at work, many women find the idea of their baby's heart being monitored electronically during labour very comforting. The baby's heartbeat is fast – twice the rate of your own – and irregular and quite an addictive sound: *'I had the belt monitor on and they said, "Do you want to take it off?" I think they always put it on when you first go into labour for fifteen minutes or so, just to check and establish what the norm is. By that stage, I had got quite used to hearing the baby's heart and I found it fascinating. That was the only intervention I had, just having the belt. I had thought I wouldn't want anything, but I did find the belt comforting . . . Listening to my baby racehorse!'*

When a baby is known to have a problem or is being born very prematurely, the mother may be particularly glad to be able to see from the digital read out on the monitor that he is all right: *'I had a lot of intervention but I didn't feel that it was unnecessary because the baby came so early. Everything I had I was glad of, even the monitor because, to me, just watching that heartbeat, knowing he was healthy, was very helpful. I needed to know; it seemed very necessary.'*

Some women, however, find watching the monitor makes them increasingly anxious that something is about to go wrong:

ADVANTAGES AND DISADVANTAGES OF ELECTRONIC MONITORING

The Advantages:

● The midwife can see clearly how your baby's heartbeat is responding to contractions

● She will be able to consult a doctor if your baby appears to be finding labour difficult

● Electronic monitoring is reassuring for many mothers, fathers and health professionals.

The Disadvantages:

● The reliability of the read-out from the monitoring machine will depend on the quality of the machine being used and on how regularly it has been serviced

● It is extremely difficult to interpret readings of a baby's heartbeat in labour. Even highly qualified and experienced midwives and doctors may disagree about what a particular reading means. A less experienced person may not notice or understand important readings

● Because of this difficulty in understanding monitor readings, some women will have emergency caesarean sections when their babies are actually perfectly all right

● Being monitored with abdominal transducers or a fetal scalp electrode often means that the mother has to stay in bed. A woman copes best with labour when she can be upright and mobile and she and her baby are much more likely to become distressed if this mobility is taken away. So monitoring may cause the distress which the machine records!

● Some parents wonder whether a fetal scalp electrode *hurts* their baby when it is clipped on. There is no answer to this question, but it's a legitimate one to ask

● Research (and there has been a lot of it) does not suggest that electronic monitoring makes labour safer for babies. Babies who are not monitored electronically do just as well. If an electronic monitor suggests that a baby is distressed, this should be confirmed by checking the baby's oxygen levels in a sample of blood taken from his scalp before any decision about doing a caesarean section is taken.

'I found it better not to watch the monitor. I just thought, "Well, what's got to happen has got to happen," and I asked for it to be turned down and I didn't look at it.'

'They monitored the baby all the way through and I got really scared at the end when I didn't understand what the monitoring meant and I thought the baby might die.'

Electronic monitoring often means that the mother is confined to bed or to a chair and being unable to move around may lead to a

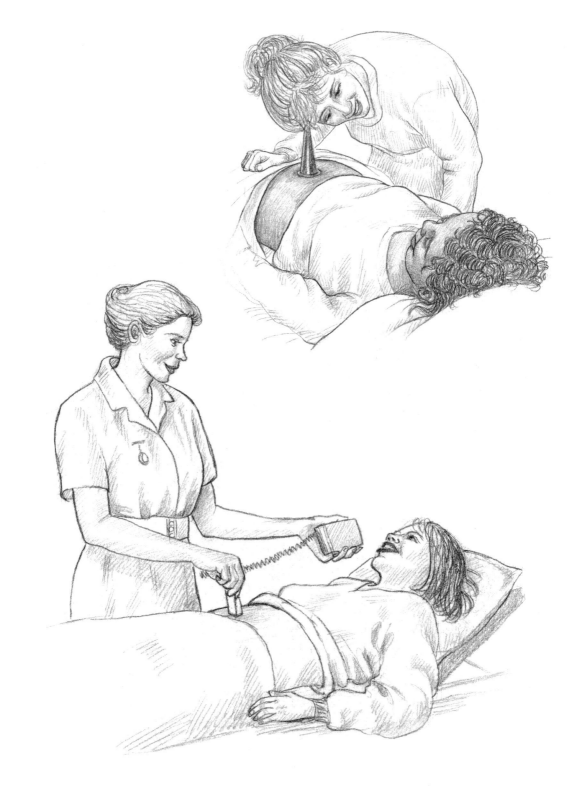

DIFFERENT KINDS OF MONITORING

There are different kinds of monitoring and you might like to think about which sort you would prefer. If you are having your baby at home, the midwife will monitor your baby's heartbeat using one of these methods:

- An ear-trumpet (Pinard's stethoscope) This is a cone-shaped piece of plastic or metal which the midwife places on your abdomen to help her listen to your baby's heartbeat with her ear

- A Hand-Held Doppler (Sonicaid) This is a kind of small ultrasound machine. The midwife places what looks like a microphone on your abdomen and you can both hear the baby's heartbeat.

If you are having your baby in hospital, you can have your baby's heartbeat monitored using either of the methods described above or in one of the following ways:

- Abdominal transducers: two round ultrasound monitors are placed on your abdomen, one at the top of your bump which is where contractions start from and one over your baby's heart. The transducers are held in place by an elastic belt. A wire from each transducer goes to a machine placed next to your chair or bed which gives a read out on paper of your baby's heartbeat and of your contractions. The midwife uses the readings to assess how well your baby is coping with labour

- Fetal scalp electrode: this is a monitor which the midwife or doctor clips onto your baby's head after your waters have broken. A wire from the monitor passes down your vagina and is attached to a machine which gives a read-out of your baby's heartbeat on paper and also a digital read out. The fetal scalp electrode may be used in conjunction with an abdominal transducer which records your contractions.

- Fetal blood sampling: the doctor or midwife can take blood from your baby's scalp during labour and analyse it to check his oxygen levels. This gives your carers more evidence on which to assess how your baby is coping with labour.

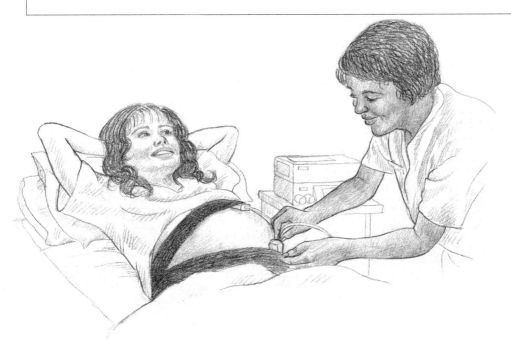

long, painful labour with the baby finally needing help in order to be born. This is another instance of the cascade of intervention mentioned earlier: *'I couldn't move around because of the monitors and I got very, very tired and it was so painful. I don't know how long I was in second stage; I remember pushing for a long time. The forceps delivery and the episiotomy were not at all what I had wanted.'*

Episiotomy

MANY PREGNANT women worry about the possibility of needing to have a cut through the back wall of the vagina during labour in order to enlarge the opening and so help the baby out. Episiotomy is the most common surgical procedure performed in this country; fortunately, there are now few hospitals where it is routinely carried out because there is no doubt that cutting this most private part of a woman's body can change the way in which she feels about herself: *'I do wish people had told me beforehand what it feels like to have had an episiotomy. I definitely don't feel the same any more. I feel different. Does everyone feel differently down below afterwards?'*

'My episiotomy healed but I can't say I'll ever be back to normal or I'll ever feel normal. I found it uncomfortable to wear jeans for a long time. Not that it hurts. It's not painful, it's just that I don't feel quite comfortable. I don't know if it's psychological, but it just doesn't feel right.'

For other women, having an episiotomy is not traumatic; how you feel may depend on your individual psychology and how sensitively you are treated: *'They had the birth plan which said I would rather not have an episiotomy but they asked if they could do a very small cut and I didn't have strong feelings about it at that point and it was fine.'*

Having an episiotomy or tearing during labour means, in most cases, that you will need to have stitches after the birth. While some women will heal quickly without any problems, for others, healing can be a long, slow process. There has been little research into how women can reduce their risk of tearing, but many women believe that massaging the perineum during pregnancy and practising pelvic floor muscle exercises will help them give birth safely:

PERINEAL MASSAGE

Although there has been little research into whether massaging the perineum (the area between the vagina and the back passage) during pregnancy helps the woman avoid a tear when she has her baby, a lot of women are convinced that it is helpful. Perineal massage is a simple technique which you carry out once a day for the last few weeks of your pregnancy.

- Use a lubricating jelly (such as KY jelly which you can get from a chemist) or an unscented oil such as almond or olive oil
- Put one finger just inside the vagina and gently move it across the rim of the vagina at the back
- After a few days, try inserting two fingers
- Eventually, you or your partner may be able to insert five fingers and open them gently until you feel a stretching sensation. When you feel this, hold the stretch for a few seconds and then let go. You can work up to several minutes of stretching and then releasing daily
- Remember that the perineum is designed by nature to stretch, but you need to encourage it to do so gradually.

'I'm doing perineal massage like crazy and I really hope it's going to help.'

'I didn't do the massage last time but I did pelvic floor muscle exercises rigorously. Learning to relax the muscles is very useful when the baby's being born. I didn't have a cut or any bruising.'

It's also important to tell your midwife if you are especially anxious to avoid an episiotomy so that she can work with you to achieve a gentle birth: *'I said to her that*

EPISIOTOMIES AND TEARS

Helping yourself avoid them

An episiotomy is a cut in the back wall of the vagina at the outlet to make the opening wider and help the baby be born more easily. Women are understandably anxious that a cut or tear affecting the vagina or the skin between the vagina and the back passage (called the perineum) will make having sex painful, or look unsightly or make using a tampon impossible. Women who have been sexually abused find the idea of a cut especially frightening because it brings back memories of the damage they have suffered to their sexual parts when they were abused.

There are things you can do to help minimise the risk of needing a cut or of tearing during labour.

- If you are upright and not sitting on your tailbone when you are pushing your baby out, your pelvis is wide open and you are giving your baby as much space as possible to find his way out easily. The easier it is for your baby to be born, the less strain he will put on your vagina and perineum
- Try and imagine your vagina opening up to allow your baby to come through easily; don't hold back
- When the midwife tells you that the baby's head will be born with the next contraction, you can go down onto all fours so that your baby's head will come out slowly from the vagina, allowing the perineum to stretch gently over his face. Such a gentle birth is excellent for your baby because it protects the delicate blood vessels inside his head from damage, and excellent for you because it minimises the risk of your perineum tearing
- The midwife will tell you to pant rather than push when your baby's head is being born and this will also help the birth to be gentle.

STITCHES AND HEALING

Many women who are having their second or subsequent babies will get through labour without tearing or needing an episiotomy; however, it is fair to say that many first-time mothers do suffer at least small tears and quite a few have an episiotomy. There are all sorts of things you can do to make life comfortable for yourself while you are healing.

● Practise your pelvic floor muscle exercises religiously – several times every day. These exercises improve the circulation to your perineum and will speed up the healing process

● Eat plenty of fibre-rich foods such as wholemeal bread, bran-based cereals, jacket potatoes, fruit with the skin on and green leafy vegetables. They will prevent you from becoming constipated and so putting strain on your stitches

● Carry a pillow with you wherever you go so that you always have something soft to sit on. If you are very sore, ask whether your midwife can get you a Valley Cushion or find out if you can hire one from your local branch of the National Childbirth Trust. This cushion is specially designed for women who have suffered tears during labour and allows you to sit comfortably without putting any pressure on your stitches

● It is *not* true that having salt baths will help your stitches heal, but they can be very soothing. If you find the salt dries your skin, try using a salt water douche: boil some water and then allow it to cool until it is comfortable to your skin. Stir in a tablespoonful of salt and then sit on the toilet and pour the salt solution between your legs from front to back so that it bathes your stitches

● If you are going to have a bath in hospital or use a hospital bidet, make sure that they are clean and if they don't look very clean, tell a member of staff but don't use them. Most postnatal infections are caught in hospitals! When using the bidet it may be more hygienic to swish the running water straight onto yourself, rather than filling the bidet and using that water

● The homeopathic remedy, Arnica, is excellent for helping heal a bruised perineum and soothing the pain of stitches.

If your stitches continue to be sore for days after the birth of your baby, be sure to let your midwife know. Don't suffer in silence; your body is too important. If when you start making love again, you find that intercourse is painful, go and see your doctor. Having one baby doesn't mean that it should be an ordeal if you want to make another!

my biggest fear was an episiotomy. I was absolutely terrified about that. I told her and she really did go out of her way to ensure that I didn't need to have one – all sorts of things like putting a hot flannel on the perineum just at the point Lucy was being born and telling me to give birth on all fours so that the baby's head would come out slowly. There are ways of avoiding interventions and I found the midwives very keen to help.'

Forceps and ventouse

SOMETIMES, EVEN though the mother has pushed as hard as she can, there are problems which mean that the birth becomes very drawn out: *'The midwife kept telling the doctors to go away and that I would be able to push this baby out without forceps. But another half hour went by and I was still pushing and the doctor came back in again and I decided that this was unbearable. In fact, the baby was stuck; the head hadn't turned.'*

In these circumstances, it is usually considered safer for the mother and for the baby if they are given some help. Often a forceps delivery means simply lifting the baby out of the vagina: *'Because Ben's head had already dropped so low, it was just a question of pulling him out the last little bit. I tried to push and take part in the birth.'*

Unless the baby needs to be born very urgently, ventouse deliveries are generally kinder for mothers than forceps because they do less damage to the vagina; you can often choose whether you would prefer to have forceps or ventouse: *'I asked to have a ventouse instead of forceps and I was lucky that the doctor who was on call was a specialist in ventouse. I just didn't fancy the metal of the forceps.'*

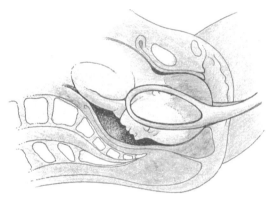

A forceps delivery

The ventouse can also be used even before the mother has started pushing in the second stage of labour: *'I had a ventouse because I had the belt monitor in the first stage and it showed that every time I had a contraction, the baby's heart rate was slowing down. I said, "Is this going to be a caesarean section?" but when they examined me, the baby's head was right there and I was fully dilated so they used the ventouse. With the second try, she was born quite quickly.'*

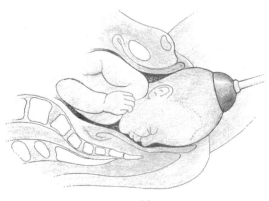

A ventouse delivery

FORCEPS AND VENTOUSE

Despite everybody's best efforts, mother's, baby's and midwife's, a baby sometimes needs extra help to be born. The mother may be exhausted after a long labour and so her contractions and pushing become weaker as the second stage of labour continues. The baby himself may have become stressed by his efforts to be born. Or he may not be in the best position to be born, and needs help to turn into a better position so that he can come into the world more easily. In all of these circumstances, the mother may be offered a forceps or a ventouse delivery to help.

Forceps come in pairs and each part has a curved blade and a handle. They are applied carefully one on either side of the baby's head and the handles fitted together. The doctor asks the mother to push when she has her next contraction and then pulls at the same time. Sometimes, the doctor needs to pull very firmly which can look rather frightening to labour supporters watching the procedure.

The ventouse looks a little like a sink plunger with a silicone plastic cup at the end. This is placed on the top of the baby's head and suction is applied either by a hand or electrical pump so that the baby's scalp is sucked into the cap. It takes six or seven minutes for the suction to take effect. The doctor can then pull the baby out of the vagina helped by the mother's own pushing efforts. Sometimes the cap comes off the baby's head and needs to be put on again.

Which should you choose?

These are some of the issues to consider:

● There are always doctors in British hospitals skilled at carrying out forceps deliveries; there may be fewer who are confident to help your baby be born by ventouse. It's a good idea to find out when you visit the hospital antenatally whether ventouse deliveries are available

● A forceps delivery can generally be carried out quite quickly and if your baby needs to be born in a couple of minutes, this is the better option. A ventouse delivery will take up to 10 minutes because time is needed for the suction to work on the baby's head

● Ventouse deliveries are far kinder for *mothers*; the suction cap takes up much less room in the vagina and causes far less damage than a pair of metal forceps. It is often not necessary to have an episiotomy with a ventouse delivery; an episiotomy is always necessary for a forceps delivery. Research suggests that as far as the baby is concerned, there may not be much to choose between forceps and ventouse, but the mother will almost certainly have much less pain and discomfort after a ventouse delivery.

Sometimes, however, the ventouse won't stay on the baby's head and then forceps are the only alternative: *'The doctor tried ventouse with me first and it kept slipping off so he said, "I'm sorry, I am going to have to use the forceps." But, as it was, Sam didn't have a mark on him afterwards.'*

CAESAREAN BIRTH

There are two kinds of caesarean section:

- Elective – this means that the mother and her obstetrician have planned and prepared for a caesarean before labour starts
- Emergency – this means that a sudden decision is made to carry out a caesarean because an unexpected problem has arisen.

Reasons for an elective caesarean

- The baby is thought to be too big to go through the mother's pelvis
- The placenta is lying across the cervix preventing the baby from getting out
- The baby is lying across the uterus rather than head or bottom down, making it impossible for him to be born vaginally
- The mother is carrying twins or triplets or more babies (although twins don't always have to be born by caesarean section)
- The baby is thought to be too weak to go through labour
- The mother has very severe pre-eclampsia and her baby needs to be born quickly both for his and for her sake
- The baby is lying in the womb in the breech position – meaning that his bottom is coming first rather than his head.

You don't have to have a caesarean if your baby is in the breech position; it's perfectly possible to give birth vaginally. However, some obstetricians are not in favour of first-time mothers having a vaginal delivery for a breech baby. You need to discuss with your midwife and consultant whether they think you should opt for a caesarean or vaginal birth and why. Remember your feelings count too. Which would you prefer?

Reasons for an emergency caesarean

- The mother has an illness, for example, diabetes, which complicates her labour
- The baby's heartbeat shows that he is not coping well with labour – the midwife and doctor describe this as the baby being 'distressed'. Another sign of distress (only sometimes) is when the waters around the baby are discoloured which means that the baby has had his bowels open in the womb; this is called having 'meconium stained waters'
- The umbilical cord comes through the cervix before the baby and is trapped between the baby's head (or bottom) and the cervix; this means that the baby's life-line is cut off
- The doctor has tried to help the baby to be born by using forceps or the ventouse, but has been unsuccessful; the only alternative is caesarean
- The cervix opens up a little but then doesn't open up any more even after many hours of labour
- After the cervix is fully open, the baby does not move down through the pelvis despite the mother's pushing; this may be because the baby does not have his head tucked closely in to his body.

These last two situations are often described as 'failure to progress' although there is no question of *failure* on either the baby's or the mother's part. Sometimes there seems to be no reason why the cervix doesn't open up fully, or why the baby isn't born in the second stage of labour. Having a problem like this in your first labour doesn't mean that it will necessarily happen again in your next.

YOUR CHOICES FOR A CAESAREAN

- Do you want to have a spinal anaesthetic, an epidural or a general anaesthetic?
- Do you want your labour supporter to stay with you throughout the operation? (This may not be possible if you are having a general anaesthetic; ask the midwife or obstetrician.)

If you are awake for the caesarean:

- Do you want the surgeon to give you a commentary on what is happening?
- Do you want to see the operation – if so, ask to have the screen removed.
- Do you want to find out the sex of your baby for yourself rather than the surgeon telling you?
- Do you want to hold your baby immediately while you are still on the operating table?
- Provided your baby is well, do you want him to stay with you until the operation is completed and afterwards, when you go to the recovery room?
- Do you want to breastfeed your baby while you are still in theatre?

If you are asleep for the operation:

- Do you want your baby to be given to your partner to hold as soon as possible?
- Do you want someone to take a photograph of your baby being born?
- Do you want your baby to be bottle-fed by the midwives during the first hours after your operation?

Emergency caesarean

WHEN YOU had expected to give birth in the normal way, it is a very frightening experience to find, in the middle of labour, that things are going wrong and that your baby needs to be born quickly by caesarean. There can be an atmosphere of panic in the delivery room with lots of people coming and going and the mother in the middle of it all desperate for the well-being of her baby:

'They put me on a drip to speed up the contractions and his heartbeat was going down and taking longer in between each contraction to recover and it was terrifying and that's when you want them to do something. I was in a real panic; the midwife was as well. She went to get the senior registrar and they were trying to get hold of the consultant and I was saying, "Get this baby out of me; just give me a caesarean; I want him out."'

Other women find that the decision to do a caesarean is taken in a calmer atmosphere which allows them to understand and appreciate what is going on: *'They did consult us all the way and kept telling us what was happening. I felt fully involved which was very positive. It wasn't like they suddenly decided to do the section and that was it.'*

'I had an emergency caesarean but the midwife explained to me what was happening. That helped me to quieten down a bit and that was very good.'

TO BE AWAKE OR NOT TO BE AWAKE?

If your baby needs to be born as soon as possible by emergency caesarean, you will probably be offered a general anaesthetic as this can be given more quickly than anything else. If you are having an elective caesarean, or you need a caesarean during labour but it's not a situation where seconds count, you can usually choose whether you want to be awake or asleep when your baby is born. Being awake means having either an epidural or a spinal anaesthetic.

Epidural/Spinal

Advantages

- You will be awake to see and hold your baby as soon as he is born; you will probably be able to cuddle him while the operation is being completed

- Your labour supporter will be able to go with you into the operating theatre and share with you the first moments of your baby's life

- Women lose less blood when they have an epidural caesarean rather than a general anaesthetic caesarean so you should recover more quickly afterwards.

Disadvantages

- Some women are terrified at the thought of being awake while they are having major surgery. If you are one of these, you will be happier having a general anaesthetic

- The noises and smells of the operating theatre can be frightening and so can the pulling and tugging sensations which you feel while your baby is being delivered.

General Anaesthetic

Advantages

- You will sleep through the whole operation and know nothing about it.

Disadvantages

- You will not be awake to greet your baby when he is born and may feel groggy for quite a few hours after the operation is finished, so it could be a while before you hold your baby for the first time

- Your partner or labour supporter will almost certainly not be able to go into the operating theatre with you

- Blood loss is greater after a general anaesthetic caesarean, so your recovery may be slower than after an epidural caesarean. There also seems to be a higher risk of having postnatal depression.

WHAT HAPPENS WHEN YOU HAVE A CAESAREAN

- Either you, or your labour supporter if you are not well enough, signs a consent form for the operation
- If this is an elective caesarean, you may be given two suppositories in your back passage a few hours before the operation to help you empty your bowels and you will be asked not to eat anything after a certain time
- The top half of the pubic area is shaved
- You put on an operating gown and any jewellery which you do not wish to take off, such as a wedding ring, is covered with tape. You are asked to wash off your make-up, remove nail varnish and take out your contact lenses or dentures if you have them
- You will probably be given a small amount of medicine to drink; this neutralises the acid in your stomach so that if any acid should pass into your lungs during the operation, they will not be damaged
- Your bladder may be emptied with a catheter (this is often done after the anaesthetic has been given so that you don't feel the midwife putting the thin plastic tube into your bladder)
- A drip is put into your arm
- You are given a general anaesthetic, a spinal, or an epidural anaesthetic. If you already have an epidural in place, this is topped up so that it is working at maximum capacity
- Women who are awake during their caesarean describe feeling strange pulling and pushing sensations in their abdomen whilst the surgeon is operating. These are not painful, but might be frightening if you're not expecting them.

Most hospitals are able to prepare a mother for a caesarean, take her to the operating theatre and deliver her baby within ten minutes of deciding that she needs to have an emergency delivery! It takes a lot longer to stitch you up again and you can expect the operation to continue for about 40 minutes after the birth of your baby.

'I had an epidural caesarean and the anaesthetist took great care to tell me exactly what he was doing and why and how I would feel.'

Elective caesarean

AN ELECTIVE caesarean is one which has been planned to take place before the woman goes into labour. Adjusting to the news that a normal delivery is not going to be possible is greatly helped by sensitive communication from health professionals: *'The consultant was very gentle and kind and reassuring. He said, "Well, I think you're going to have to see this baby a bit sooner than you'd expected." We talked about how quickly I needed to have the caesarean and he came up to the ward to see me and the baby afterwards and I thought that was really good.'*

WHAT TO EXPECT AFTER A CAESAREAN

The first few days after the caesarean:

- You may have a lot of pain. Ask for an injection or tablets to control the pain for as long as you need them. You now have a tiny baby to get to know and care for and *enjoy*. You can't do any of these things if you are in pain
- You will not be allowed to have anything to eat or drink for quite a while after your operation. The drip in your arm ensures that you do not become dehydrated. Many women feel ravenously hungry after the birth of their baby and find waiting until they can have a snack very hard
- A physiotherapist will visit you soon after your operation and show you how to cough to keep your chest clear, and also how to get out of bed and walk around. Despite your worst fears, you will not split in half, and the more mobile you can be, the less likely you are to have problems
- For a day or two after the operation, you may have a catheter in your bladder and/or a drain coming from your wound and emptying into a bottle. Having to take a catheter bag and drainage bottle with

you wherever you go is a bit complicated, but it's still important to try to get up and around

- A midwife will show you how to hold your baby or lie with him beside you so that you can feed him without hurting your abdomen. It is perfectly possible to breastfeed your baby after a caesarean. You can be prescribed painkillers which will not harm him if they are absorbed into your milk
- And how will you *feel* after your caesarean? Some women just feel very, very happy that their baby has been safely born. Some may be going through an anxious and lonely time because their baby is in Special Care, and some who have their baby with them feel unhappy and disappointed that they were not able to give birth vaginally. All these feelings are normal and to be respected. You might find it helpful, if you are feeling unhappy or even if you're not, to talk to your midwife about the caesarean and why it was necessary, and to share your feelings with your partner or friends.

Nowadays, many women choose to have an epidural anaesthetic for their caesarean so that they can be awake to greet their baby when he is born and so that their labour supporter can be with them. While it is not always possible to choose between an epidural and a general anaesthetic if you need an emergency caesarean – in the vast majority of cases, you can certainly choose to have an epidural if your caesarean is an elective one: *'I had an epidural for the caesarean. Phil was with me and after the baby was born, we held her together while they sewed me up.'*

If the woman is not able to hold her baby herself as soon as he is born, she can see her partner or labour supporter holding him: *'He was with*

COPING WITH PAIN AFTER A CAESAREAN

During the first 48 hours you will be offered a range of pain relief which may include:

- Intramuscular injections (given in your bottom or thigh) of pethidine, omnopon or a similar pain-relieving drug (These drugs are safe to take if you are breast-feeding as only a very small amount passes to your baby in your milk.)

or

- Epidural top-ups if you have had your caesarean under epidural anaesthesia

or

- A pump filled with a pain-relieving drug attached to a drip in your arm. You operate the pump yourself so that you can control your own pain-relief. This is called Patient Controlled Analgesia or PCA.

After 48 hours you will probably change to:

- Pain-killing tablets such as paracetamol
  or
- You may like to use your TENS machine if you have one. The midwife or physiotherapist will show you where to apply the pads.

THE IMPORTANT POINT IS:
Don't be afraid to ask for more pain-killers if you want them. You mustn't be prevented from cuddling and feeding your baby because of pain. Ask for another injection or more tablets *before* the pain becomes intolerable so that you keep yourself always comfortable.

me when I had the section and ended up holding the baby first which was really good; it was lovely.'

Finding out why you needed a caesarean

A CAESAREAN section is a major piece of abdominal surgery and most women will need several weeks and often months to recover from it. There is little doubt that a woman recovers more easily if her mind is at rest because she knows why her caesarean was necessary and whether, should she decide to have another baby, she will need a caesarean next time as well. The effects of not knowing the reason for the caesarean can be ongoing anxiety and distress: 'A lot of the feelings about the caesarean came long afterwards – and now it's still a problem for me. What on earth was going on?'

It is, therefore, very important that the mother doesn't go home with her new baby without receiving a thorough explanation: 'I asked to go through my notes so that I knew exactly why I'd needed the section and the midwife was very helpful. She went through the notes with a fine-tooth comb; that was really important.'

Sometimes, sadly, it seems to be impossible to get the information you need: 'I asked a junior doctor about seeing my notes as I was interested in why they'd actually done the caesarean because I didn't know what had happened and he said, "Oh that's not possible; you'll have to write to the hospital

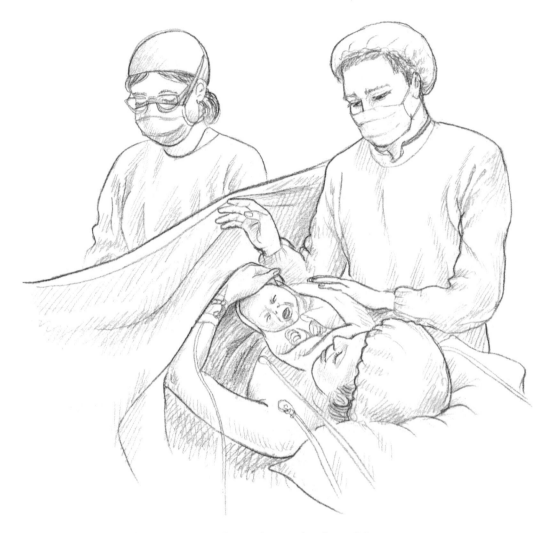

administrator." I said, "I'm not attacking what you've done, I just want to know", but they wouldn't tell me.'

In such a case, it is worth plucking up your courage and asking a more senior doctor or the midwife who was with you during labour if either of them can discuss the caesarean with you. You are legally entitled to see your notes and if you have any difficulties obtaining information, ask to speak to the Director of Midwifery Services. In many places, the Director will visit mothers at home to sort out any problems.

Understanding what happened during labour and the events lead-

CARING FOR YOURSELF AFTER A CAESAREAN

- **Getting out of bed** — Curl your body so both knees come up to your chest. Then roll carefully into a sitting position at the edge of the bed so you can get off. Midwives will help you.

- **Sitting in bed or in a chair** — Use several pillows to make yourself as comfortable as possible, especially when you are feeding your baby. Use the bell to call for help if you find it difficult to lift your baby out of the cot.

- **Protecting your scar** — Support your scar with a pillow or your hands when you cough, sneeze or laugh.

- **Coping with wind** — Many women say that the worst aspect of a caesarean is the wind you suffer from afterwards. Drinking peppermint cordial seems to help as does walking about.

- **Underwear** — High-waisted knickers are the most comfortable as they keep the pressure off your wound. Try men's boxer shorts or NCT 'string-vest' knickers.

- **Shoes** — Slip on slippers are the easiest, as it may be hard to bend down to do up laces.

- **When home...** — Have nappy-changing things downstairs and also somewhere for the baby to sleep so that you don't have to keep going upstairs with him.

- **Getting help** — Line up emergency help for when you get home – friends, family, anyone. Get your visitors working. Ask guests to make tea, put washing out etc. Try to avoid lifting and driving – it is recommended that you don't drive for up to four weeks after the operation.

ing up to the decision to do the operation help the woman to feel good about the way in which her baby was born and about herself:

'I didn't feel disappointed because I knew exactly why it had happened.'

'People's first reaction when they hear you've had a section is, "Oh no; that's a real shame", but I'm saying, "No, no; it's not a shame; I know it had to be that way and he's here and he's fine and it's OK."'

CASCADE OF INTERVENTION

Sometimes, intervention in labour leads to more intervention, precipitating a cascade. This chart suggests one possible sequence of events:

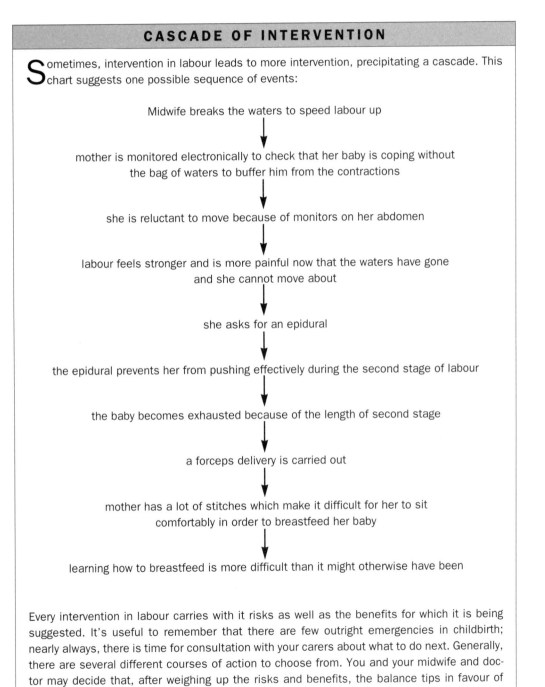

Midwife breaks the waters to speed labour up

↓

mother is monitored electronically to check that her baby is coping without the bag of waters to buffer him from the contractions

↓

she is reluctant to move because of monitors on her abdomen

↓

labour feels stronger and is more painful now that the waters have gone and she cannot move about

↓

she asks for an epidural

↓

the epidural prevents her from pushing effectively during the second stage of labour

↓

the baby becomes exhausted because of the length of second stage

↓

a forceps delivery is carried out

↓

mother has a lot of stitches which make it difficult for her to sit comfortably in order to breastfeed her baby

↓

learning how to breastfeed is more difficult than it might otherwise have been

Every intervention in labour carries with it risks as well as the benefits for which it is being suggested. It's useful to remember that there are few outright emergencies in childbirth; nearly always, there is time for consultation with your carers about what to do next. Generally, there are several different courses of action to choose from. You and your midwife and doctor may decide that, after weighing up the risks and benefits, the balance tips in favour of intervention. Or you may decide otherwise.

ASKING QUESTIONS

IF THERE's one theme that tends to run through all that the women have said in this chapter, it is the importance of understanding what is happening in labour and of having good lines of communication with the medical and midwifery staff. The result of not knowing what is going on is increased stress for the woman and therefore a far greater likelihood of things going wrong during the birth:

'They told me that I was going to have an emergency caesarean and that they couldn't wait for my husband to arrive and they didn't tell me anything that was happening or whether I'd be awake or asleep. And I started shaking, just shaking. I couldn't stop myself and a doctor said to me, "What's the matter?" and I said, "I think I'm terrified."'

If a woman is given an honest and straightforward explanation of why an intervention is needed by someone whom she has grown to trust, the intervention becomes much more acceptable even if it is something she would very much like to have avoided:

'The midwife explained very carefully that if I didn't have an episiotomy, she thought I would have a bad tear, and so I agreed with her to go ahead.'

Generally in labour, it is perfectly possible for the woman and her carers to reach a compromise which is satisfactory to both of them; in the following example the mother felt that she was still in control of her labour and the professionals felt that their advice was being respected: *'I think they are open to compromise as well. I asked for more time in second stage because I wanted to see if the contractions would sort themselves out and get started again. They said, "OK, let's wait another twenty minutes", and I thought, "That's very sensible."'*

So don't be afraid to ask; being psychologically healthy and happy after the birth is as important as being physically well.

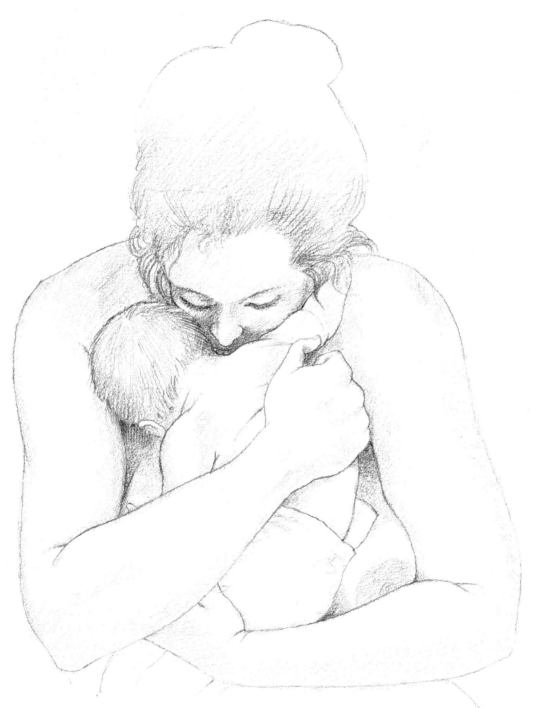

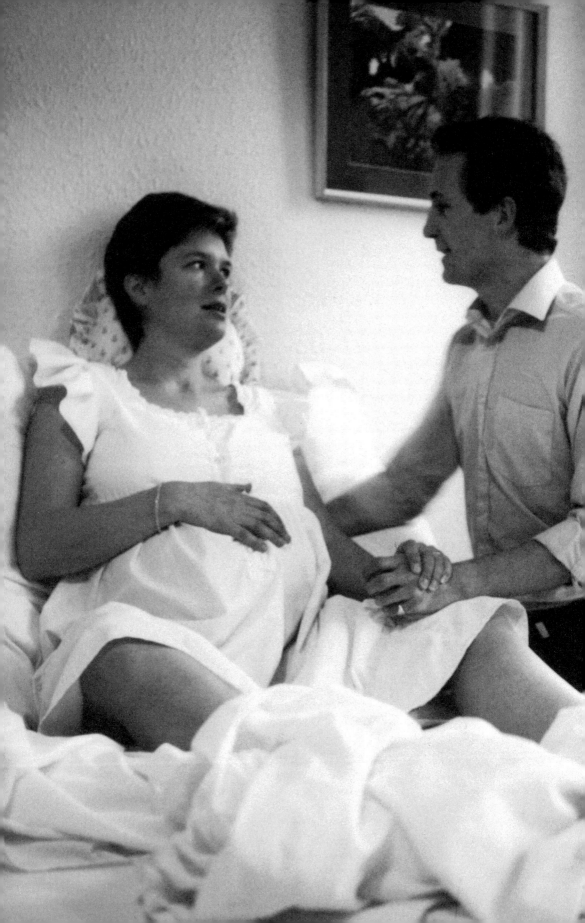

CHAPTER *seven* Labour supporters

NO TWO LABOURS are the same. If you have already had a baby, what happened to you during your first labour is certainly not guaranteed to repeat itself next time round, although there may be similarities. If you're about to experience your first labour, you have no blue print to which you can refer to give you an idea of how things might go. This uncertainty makes up a large part of the nervousness which women facing labour feel.

If you think back to childhood, the thing which you probably used to find most helpful when you had something difficult to do was asking your best friend to come along with you. Having someone's hand to hold, and someone to support you who was on your side helped you find the courage to face up to difficult tasks. As adults, we often have to confront challenges on our own and we accept this as part of the process of growing up. However, labour is one occasion when you can still choose to have someone with you who is part of your everyday life, whom you know well and who is there entirely to support you. Whether you are having your baby at home or in hospital, a labour supporter is likely to help you relax and to increase your enjoyment of the birth.

There has been a lot of research into the usefulness of labour supporters and the results have often been staggering. A supporter can influence the events of the labour itself and also how the woman feels about her labour afterwards. Studies have shown that women who are supported during labour need to have fewer pain-killers, experience fewer interventions and give birth to stronger babies. After their babies are born, supported women feel better about themselves, their labours and their babies!

LABOUR SUPPORTER'S ROLE

Research suggests that there is nothing more effective in helping a woman cope well with labour than good support from her midwife and chosen labour companion. Loving support reduces a woman's need for pain-killing drugs and medical interventions in labour, and increases her satisfaction with her birth experience.

So how can you help?

- Perhaps most importantly, you need to help the mother get comfortable during labour. If she wants to stand or kneel or sit or lie on her side, help her to do so and then help her to change her position when she becomes uncomfortable again. If she is kneeling, she might like a pillow under her knees and under her ankles; if she is sitting astride a chair, she might like a pillow across the back of the chair to lean on. If she is standing, she might like to lean onto you and you can rock with her from side to side. She might like to squat down between your legs if you are sitting on a chair, and lean on your thighs

- A woman needs to be loved and touched during labour; although she may push you away one moment, she will almost certainly want a hug the next! Tell her she's wonderful because when labour gets tough and a woman begins to feel that she's not coping well, it is tremendously helpful to her to know that you appreciate the effort she is making and believe in her

- The mother may be trying to help herself through contractions by concentrating on keeping her breathing even; if her shoulders become hunched and tense, her breathing is likely to become panicky. You can help by leaning gently on her shoulders so that they drop down and her breathing relaxes. She might like you to breathe through contractions with her, keeping eye contact with her and encouraging her to copy you as you breathe calmly in through your nose and blow out gently through your mouth

- Information is vital to help the mother relax (and to help you relax as well.) What a labouring woman most needs to know is whether her baby is okay. You can ask the midwife the questions which the mother may not be in a fit state to ask herself and then pass the information on to her. She will hear and understand what you say better than what the midwife says.

FATHERS

YEARS AGO IN this country, a woman who was having a baby would always have had other women to support her – probably her mother, her sister, a friend, or all of these. Birth was a time when women rallied round and gave each other the support which it was felt that women were best able to give because of their natural rapport with a

USEFUL THINGS FOR LABOUR SUPPORTERS TO HAVE READY

- *Drinks and snacks* (for you and the mother) – sandwiches, nuts and raisins, fruit and chocolate, orange or lemon squash are possibilities; avoid strong-smelling or highly flavoured foods which might make the mother feel sick

- *Ice-cubes* – if you are going to hospital, put the cubes in a wide-topped thermos flask. They're wonderful for the mother to suck between contractions. You may enjoy them as well!

- *Socks and a warm shawl* – especially towards the end of the first stage of labour, the mother may feel very cold and want the comfort of a shawl to put round her shoulders or socks to warm her feet

- *Unscented vegetable oil* – for massaging the mother's back or shoulders

- *Small natural sponge* – this can be soaked in iced water for the mother to suck between contractions, or you can use it to wipe her face gently. A natural sponge has

a far more pleasant texture than a synthetic one

- *Soft face flannel* – for you to give to the mother to wipe her face, neck and hands

- *Tapes and cassette player* – so that you and the mother can listen to music to help you relax during labour. (Check with the hospital that you are allowed to use a mains-powered cassette player on the premises.)

- *PP3 batteries* – if the mother wants to use a TENS machine to help her cope with contractions. Make sure that you have spare batteries in case you need more at 3am when it's impossible to buy them!

- *Camera and film* – to take lots of photos of the new baby!

- *Small change for the telephone* – so that you can spread the good news after the birth of the baby!

woman in labour. It was almost unheard of for a man to be with his wife during labour even though virtually every woman gave birth at home. In many cultures in the world today, it is still true that the only witnesses of labour and birth are women.

When, in the 1960s and 70s, women in the UK started more and more to have their babies in hospital, traditional sources of support were no longer available to them. Hospitals did not want the women who might once have offered their help to a friend or relative in labour; they were strictly the territory of health professionals. Support during labour was provided as far as possible by the midwife but she might well have several women in her care and her attention could not be given entirely to one person. Nor was she necessarily a

LABOUR SUPPORTERS NEED TO LOOK AFTER THEMSELVES

- Remember that labour wards are hot, and even if the mother is giving birth at home, you will still get hot as you will be working hard to support her. Wear a t-shirt or open-necked shirt, or loose clothes. If you become overheated, you will start to feel faint and it will not be helpful either to the mother or the midwife if you pass out!

- Just as the mother needs food in early labour and lots of drinks as labour progresses, so do you. There's no shame in having a snack if you need one; you will be better able to support the mother if you are not weak from hunger

- You might need to have a short time away from the mother every now and then; it is enormously stressful being with someone who is going through a traumatic and painful experience. If you want to leave the room for a few minutes, do so; the midwife will care for the mother until you return and will also fetch you if necessary!

- Your need to know and understand what is happening during the labour is every bit as great as the mother's. Ask all the questions you want and establish a good relationship with the midwife so that she consults you as well as the mother about decisions regarding the management of the labour

- After the baby is born, you need to talk to someone about what happened during the labour, how you felt, and how you feel now. Mothers need to debrief their labours, but so do those who have supported them. It is often easier for women to find other people who will listen to them talk about their birth experiences than it is for supporters, especially if the supporters are men. Try and think of someone to whom you can turn.

familiar face to the labouring woman. The fact that the midwife had clinical responsibilities meant that she was perceived by the woman as being part of the hospital establishment rather than as someone who was there simply to support her.

During the 1970s, women's organisations began to campaign for fathers to be allowed to stay with their partners during labour. The need to provide women with support during labour coincided with men beginning to insist on having a greater share in family life. The natural extension of men's new-found role as actively involved members of the family as opposed to being merely remote breadwinners, was to assist at the birth of their children. It was not an easy task to change the hospital system so that fathers who had traditionally been fiercely barred from the delivery room would be made welcome there. But the campaign was overwhelmingly successful and the situation today is such that fathers are *expected* to be present at the birth of their babies. Indeed, there may now be too much pressure on men to support their partners in labour when some fathers feel that this is a role they cannot take on.

A lot of men, however, are glad to be present, although research suggests that most do not take an active part in labour but are simply there as onlookers. This is understandable; perhaps for the first time in their lives, a man who is attending the birth of his child is entering into a woman's world. He may have a limited

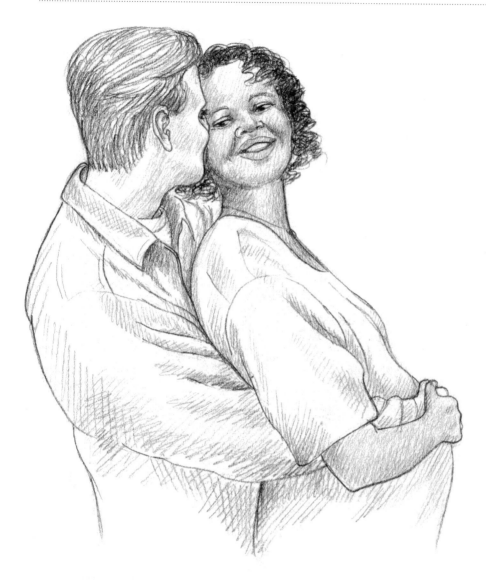

understanding of the process of birth; he may be frightened and distressed by his partner's pain; he may not like seeing her behave in ways
she would not normally behave; he may be upset by the sight of
blood. On top of all this, he has to cope with the tremendous change
in his own life which is taking place during labour: just as his partner
is becoming a mother, so he is becoming a father. It is difficult to be
single-minded in supporting another person when one's own emotions are in a state of turmoil.

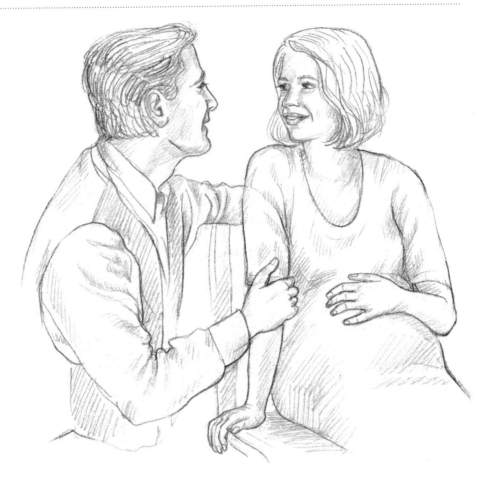

Despite all of this, men seem to meet their partners' expectations very satisfactorily during labour as these women will confirm:

'It's someone there whom you know very well and who can talk to you and take your mind off it. And he understood what I was on about.'

'My husband was there although he did nothing at all apart from carry my bag and sit and watch. He didn't say anything to me, but he was very reassuring and very calm. Having him there just a few yards away made it all better. I think I would have coped less well if I'd been on my own even though, looking back, there's nothing quantifiable that he did.'

'It's important to have someone that you love there.'

'I wouldn't want anyone else to see me in that situation. I've got a friend who is a midwife and I was wondering beforehand whether I would like her with me, and I don't think I would because I wouldn't want her to see me in that situation whereas I felt quite happy with Sam. I mean Sam has seen me at my worst and I took it for granted that he would be there and I wouldn't have wanted anyone else.'

Many women will report how immediate was the effect on their labour if their partner left the room: *'When Brett went out, just for a minute, to go to the toilet or something, the contractions were a lot worse because he wasn't there.'*

When labour is complicated or a caesarean section is necessary, it's not possible for the father to *do* anything except to be with the woman, but his presence is, in these circumstances, even more critically important: *'Sanjoy being there during the operation was really important because it was very frightening to go through that. He was a real support; he was telling me what was going on and he was marvellous.'*

Sometimes men are not allowed to stay in the delivery room when medical procedures or internal examinations are being performed; this can be very distressing for the woman and is perhaps a case where you might want to be assertive and ask the reason for your partner being sent out: *'I don't understand why they sent Ian out when I was having my epidural because that was the time I needed him the most, that was the time it was hurting the most. I was completely on my own and panic set in. At least if you've got somebody there, they can hold your hand and look at you and tell you everything's going to be all right.'*

There are a variety of helpful things which men can do if they feel able to be more involved with the labour than merely observing it:

'He was very useful because he kept taking me to the loo which was good because I felt scared about going on my own.'

'He kept saying, "You're doing really well; come on, you're doing really well."'

'My husband was a great support, rubbing my back, just firm pressure in the small of my back.'

'If ever I was losing myself, he'd say: "Just concentrate, concentrate."'

The father can also act as an advocate for the woman, explaining to staff what she wants: *'Even when I'd been given diamorphine, he was still being strong about what we wanted to happen and was trying to fight my corner for me. He would say, "Well, I don't think this is what we want to happen here", or, "Could you explain why you want to do that to her?" Although I was pretty out of it at this stage, he was still very much stating what our position was, so he was very supportive.'*

Some men are natural labour supporters and seem to know instinctively how to help: *'He would say, "Get ready with your gas and air now", as he could see the contraction building. The two of us were really working together. Absolutely brilliant.'*

When the father doesn't want to be there

SOME MEN definitely do not want to be present at the birth of their baby, and some women consider that their partner would not be helpful: *'My partner missed the birth because they took me in to be induced and then it happened so quickly. But looking back on it, I'm so glad he wasn't there because he'd been with me when they gave me the Prostin gel and he'd kept saying, "Ooh, I don't like this." I think I dealt with the labour very well but if I'd had to think about him as well, I'm not sure what would have happened. They took blood from the baby's head at one stage and it was traumatic for me, but I think if he'd been there, watching, it would have been awful. We both agree that what we want next time is for him to come in just after the birth.'*

Birth is the outcome of the sexual act and is itself a sexual experience involving the most intimate parts of the woman's body. For some men, seeing their partner exposed to the gaze of a midwife (possibly a male midwife) and perhaps of male doctors, is profoundly upsetting. Witnessing their partner's pain and perhaps seeing the woman's sexual organs damaged during the birth can give rise to feelings of guilt and have a long-term effect on their sex lives:

'Steve doesn't want to be present for the birth and I agree. The last birth had dramatic effects on our sex life which was non-existent for a long while and I think part of it was that he watched me and saw me doing things I don't normally do and behaving in a way I don't normally behave. And he saw me being snipped and stitched and it's quite a lot for him to have watched. I think it left him feeling inadequate, that he couldn't do anything to help. He felt that if he hadn't had sex with me, I wouldn't have been going through that.'

It is almost certainly very unhelpful if a man agrees to be present during labour when he really doesn't want to be; the decision as to whether or not he should be present needs to be a mutual one. And it's still possible – even with today's pressures – for a couple to decide that the father will *not* be present; he can often be helping out elsewhere in the family: *'We've agreed that as he doesn't particularly feel the need to be there, he'll look after our little girl while I'm giving birth.'*

Fathers' experiences

A MAN'S EXPERIENCE of pregnancy, labour and early parenthood mirrors the woman's in so far as it is often made up of a great deal of anxiety and uncertainty as well as pride and excitement. Although his life is undergoing as radical a change as hers, he may receive much less support than she does and much less recognition from others that something major is happening to him. Yet, when fathers talk about labour, it is clear that they have to ride on the same emotional rollercoaster as do their partners. The time spent waiting for labour to start can be highly charged:

'She started having very mild contractions; I couldn't sleep because I didn't want to miss out on anything. Then the contractions stopped. There were several days of "is she/isn't she?" which I found emotionally draining.'

'Anticipating the labour was almost unbearable.'

When labour finally gets underway, the father's feelings are probably exactly the same as the mother's: *'I felt a mixture of relief that the labour had started and terror at what was going to happen.'*

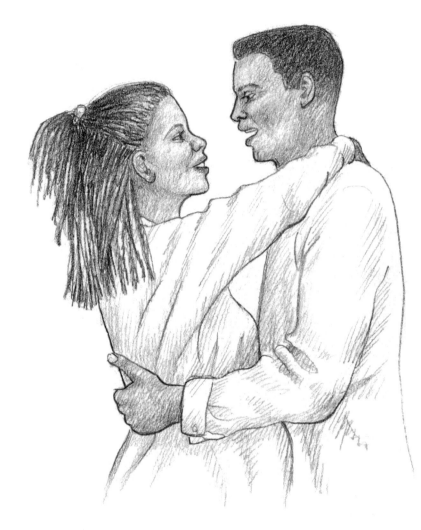

Many men enjoy having a part to play during the labour. Doing something distracts from the worry about whether the labour is progressing normally and helps them cope with their partner's pain:

'I did some back massage to help her through the contractions. I wanted to be involved; I wanted to be needed – and loved – as well.'

But often, a father may feel that there is nothing he can do, and while the woman is totally focused on her contractions, he is left to cope with the intensity of his own emotions, as these three men describe:

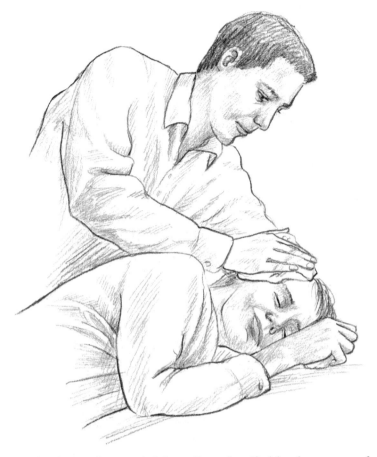

'For the last few hours of Monica's labour, I was horrified by the amount of pain she was going through.'

'At times, I felt physically sick from worry.'

'All I could do during the really difficult parts was talk, swallow hard and admire her courage as she pushed the baby out.'

Guilt that they are partly the cause of the woman's suffering is often to the fore in fathers' minds: *'When I remember what Janette went through, I feel very uncomfortable talking about the birth.'*

And for some men the experience of being present during their partner's labour is one which they do not look back on with any satisfaction: '*To be honest, it was probably one of the most unpleasant experiences of my life.*'

The moment of birth can be overwhelming – matching the intensity of the mother's emotions in combining joy at the arrival of the baby with relief that labour is safely over, as these two new fathers testify:

'*I cried and cried and my whole body ached. I was so relieved that the baby was absolutely fine and that Henna was absolutely fine.*'

'*Before the birth, I had not thought about holding him. The midwife gave him to me and he was so alive – looking at me – and so innocent.*'

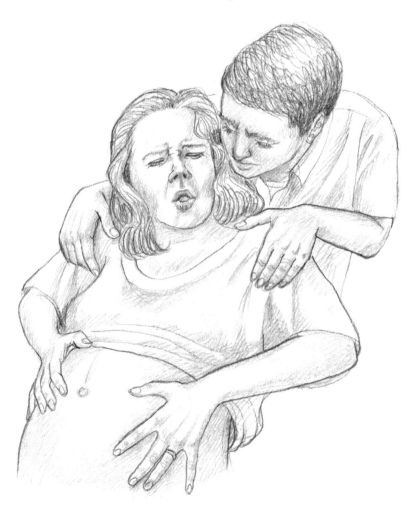

OTHER LABOUR SUPPORT

SOME WOMEN choose to have both their partner and a woman supporter with them in labour. There is excellent research to show how effective a woman supporter can be in improving the outcome of labour and in helping the mother to feel confident about taking up the responsibilities of caring for her new baby. In some parts of the country, it is now possible for a pregnant woman to employ a 'doula' or female labour supporter. The two get to know each other during the last weeks of the pregnancy; the doula then supports the mother through labour and visits her in hospital or at home afterwards to help her with babycare tasks and to adjust emotionally to becoming a parent.

Generally, however, if a mother chooses to have a female supporter with her, it is someone who is related to her or who has been a friend for a long time:

'I'd like my sister or a very close friend to be there as well. Your partner can have a break because they can take it in turns to look after you; also having another woman is different from a man. Maybe she can empathise a bit better with what's going on.'

'My instinctive feeling is to have women around me so I'll have a friend staying in the house to look after me.'

One obvious choice for some women is their mother, particularly if you get on well: *'My mum was brilliant. She's got this personality about her of "You can do it. Let's do it right." I don't know if it's because she's been*

CHECKLIST FOR LABOUR SUPPORTERS
P OSITION
Is the mother changing her position regularly and moving about?
U RINATION
Are you reminding her to go to the toilet every hour?
R ELAXATION
Is she as relaxed as possible?
R ESPIRATION
Is she breathing evenly, and not gasping?
R EST
Is she making the most of the break between contractions to rest and refresh herself?
R EASSURANCE
Are you giving her constant encouragement and reassurance?

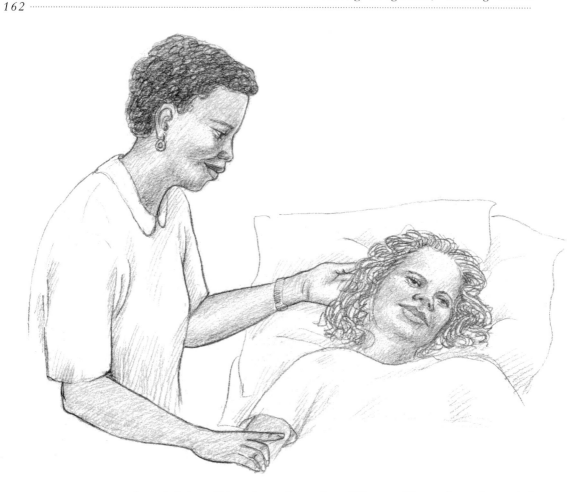

through it herself, but she really made a difference. She made good, practical suggestions and was just so positive.'

'During the actual birth, Johnny was there and I found that very comforting but it was my sister I hung onto. I tried to lean on Johnny but he was too tall and I couldn't get comfortable. She was just the right height and it was a lot easier.'

At home, you can choose to have whoever you want present for the birth. Most hospitals are equally flexible although some may prefer that you have only one person. It's really important for you to think carefully about who is going to be with you as the person or people whom you choose as labour supporters will certainly affect how you feel about your labour afterwards, and may influence what happens

DOULAS

'Doula' is a Greek word. A doula is a woman who has herself given birth and brought up children and whose job is to help other women give birth and to teach them how to care for their babies.

How do doulas help women in labour? What the research shows.

In the 1980s, three doctors working in the large maternity hospital in Guatemala City decided to see whether women would have shorter labours if they had someone to support them. At the time, it was not allowed for women labouring at this hospital to have companions with them during labour and they were left on their own by the midwives until just before their babies were born. Their labours tended to be very long. The doctors recruited women who were themselves mothers to come into the hospital as labour supporters or 'doulas'. The doulas were instructed to do nothing more than hold the woman who was in labour, talk to her, massage her, encourage her, and stay with her until her baby was born. By this simple means, the average length of labour was reduced for women having their first babies from 19 hours to 8 hours! Women who had doulas allocated to them were far less likely to need a caesarean section or a forceps delivery than women who had no one to support them. They also gave birth to healthier babies. Since this famous study was carried out, it has been shown that, not only in Third World countries, but also in affluent Western countries where the standard of care in hospitals is much higher, women still have fewer complications in labour and their babies are born healthier if they are supported by a doula. After the birth, women who have had doula support feel good about their labours and form a close relationship with their babies very quickly. It would appear that being 'mothered' whilst in labour helps a woman to become a satisfied mother herself.

Why can't midwives be doulas?

Many, perhaps all midwives would like to be doulas. They see their role as supporting the woman in labour by responding to her physical and emotional needs. However, midwives are often very busy people even if they are only caring for one woman and in many hospitals, each midwife will have several women in labour under her care. This 'busy-ness' may prevent the midwife from simply staying close to the mother, holding and comforting her, noticing her changes of mood and offering her the small physical comforts which make labour easier. It is probably more possible for a midwife to offer the kind of support a doula offers if the mother is giving birth at home, but even here, she still has to make sure that health authority regulations are obeyed, that certain procedures are carried out at certain times and that records are carefully kept.

Would it be economic to employ doulas?

Marsden Wagner of the World Health Organisation has calculated that the United States could save US$1000m a year if doulas were employed to support women in labour. This figure is based on research which has shown that far fewer women have forceps or ventouse deliveries or caesarean sections when they are supported by doulas, and that fewer of their babies need to be looked after in Special Care Baby Units.

during it. If you already have children, you might like to consider whether you want them to be present at the birth: '*My three-year-old daughter was with me during most of the labour – it felt so* right *that she should be there.*'

Although adults are often anxious that small children will be upset if they see their mother in pain, and will be frightened by the sounds she makes and the sight of blood, research suggests that they take it all in their stride. Some studies have found that children who are present at the birth of a sibling have a special relationship with him or her. Women who choose to have their children with them are emphasising that birth is, for them, a family affair: '*Robin was giving me cuddles between contractions. He was very supportive and not at all bothered by my contractions. When the baby was being born, he stroked my shoulder and when the baby's head came out, he said, "Baby . . . baby." When she was born, I was crying but he knew somehow that I wasn't sad. I think the fact that he was there helped us to bond as a family.*'

MIDWIVES AS SUPPORTERS

MIDWIVES ARE special people who come into your life for a relatively short period of time but who can make a profound impact on it. It is essential to have a good relationship with the midwife who is caring for you in labour, so that you feel able to trust her advice and know that she will not do anything without taking your opinion and feelings into account first. It is precisely because the support which a woman receives from her midwife in labour is so crucial that the maternity services are being reorganised and, within the next five years, every woman should be reasonably sure of knowing the midwife who will help her to give birth. Up until now, this has generally not been the case because women often see a different midwife at each clinic visit and walk into the delivery suite at the hospital not knowing who is going to look after them. The consequences of meeting different professionals at every antenatal visit, and of seeing yet more doctors and midwives during and after the birth can be very negative: '*I saw about eight different midwives in hospital and different doctors and I found it all so confusing. They were all telling me to do different things. This was especially so after the birth.*'

There are now many schemes which enable women to get to know just a small group of midwives who are responsible for all their care, or even to choose to be cared for by a particular midwife. You can certainly ask whether such a scheme is running in your area, as these three women did:

'I actually had the midwife who I've booked with this time for my last labour. She was the one I wanted and we've looked at my notes and talked about what I want.'

'I asked for one specific midwife. I'm quite nervous anyway and I want the chance to form a relationship with her. Although a birth plan is a nice idea – if you've never been pregnant before, it's very idealistic. It's all right putting things down but you don't know what labour's going to be like at the time. I've talked through my ideas with the midwife.'

'I think if I hadn't had the midwife I knew, my birth might have turned out very different. She was so considerate of my views because of the trust that we had built up between us.'

Women explain how the best midwives are the ones who have confidence in you, who offer both physical and emotional support, who keep you always informed and respect your opinions, and who quite clearly care about you and want what is best for you:

'My midwife was super. She never ever gave out any negative vibes; she was always positive.'

'A community midwife popped into the room and she was a wonderful lady who literally hugged me and she was undoubtedly the best physical support I had. She was wonderful; she was a big-busted lady with a bright red t-shirt and I just know that I was literally hugged while I was pushing and it was wonderful.'

'The midwife was supportive and reassuring and told me what was going on.'

'It's good that the midwife who'd been with me in labour came with me when I went to have a caesarean – a familiar face.'

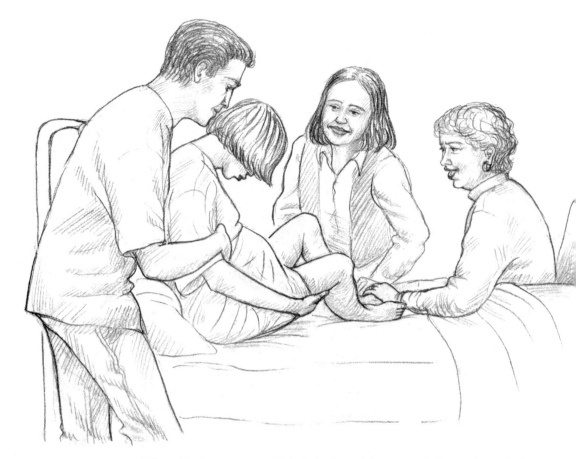

'The midwives – you couldn't fault them. They consulted me, they asked me what I wanted, they explained everything.'

'The midwives came to see me on the ward afterwards which was lovely. They took an interest; they cared.'

If a woman is unsure about how her partner will cope during labour, she may be relieved to know that the midwife will try to look after him as well as her: *'I know my husband will feel better if it's not all left up to him. He's fairly tough but he'll still feel a bit upset and anxious seeing me in pain, so he'll be glad if the midwife's behind him telling him what to do.'* Midwives don't have to take over from labour supporters; they can simply show them how to be helpful to the woman: *'She advised Tom to do back massage which really helped and it was wonderful to have someone there who was helping us both through it.'*

Not having a midwife in whom she feels confident has just the same effect on a woman as sensing that her partner doesn't really want to be with her in labour. She becomes increasingly anxious and labour becomes more difficult. Midwives do not always provide quality care if they have to look after a woman whose way of handling labour they find embarrassing, or if they are working in an environment where they do not feel confident:

'The next couple of hours are a bit of a blur. At eight o'clock, the midwife suggested that I try using the Entonox. I'm not sure why because I didn't want it, but I didn't question. I think I didn't question because I was constantly aware that the midwife wasn't very relaxed and I didn't want to do anything to make her worse. I can remember trying to crack jokes between contractions just to improve the atmosphere. I think she wanted me to be a "good patient" and I wanted to be able to relax and be just a woman in labour.'

'Not all midwives are sensitive. In second stage, she was saying to me, "Breathe! Breathe!" And I was obviously breathing. I was making a lot of noise and was coping really well. Later when the midwife was doing the stitching, I said I was going to shout and as soon as I made a sound, the midwife backed off – she couldn't handle the noise at all. She was not comfortable with women using noise to cope with pain.'

The moment when a woman perceives that her midwife or labour companion are doubting her ability to give birth can be the lowest point in her labour. One of the main themes which runs through women's accounts of how they were supported in labour relates to whether their midwife and chosen supporter had, or did not have, confidence in them: *'I heard at one stage the midwife whispering to a doctor who was passing in the corridor, "Yes, she's pushing but she can't make it," and I thought, "Oh God: I'm going to have a caesarean". To me, to realise that the midwife and Chris as well were saying, "She can't do it", was a desperate moment; it was incredibly stressful. That's when I was ready to give up.'* *'You can appear to be almost totally unconscious or in another world, but you're still extremely sensitive to the little signs that indicate that people are losing heart.'*

When the woman's carers have confidence in her and demonstrate it, even a woman who is terrified of giving birth can be powered through her labour: '*My midwife kept telling me that I could do it because I kept saying that I couldn't do it, that I was quite incapable of doing it, that I couldn't cope. She kept saying, "You are coping, you are doing it", and I kept asking for every form of pain relief I'd ever heard of and she kept saying, "No – you can do it without; you can do it with just gas and air". And I did! She was right and because I had no confidence that I could do it, she helped me tremendously.*'

Such carers do more for the woman than helping her achieve a successful delivery; they can influence how she feels about herself for the rest of her life. They can transmit their own confidence to her so that she takes up her new role as a mother feeling on top of the world.

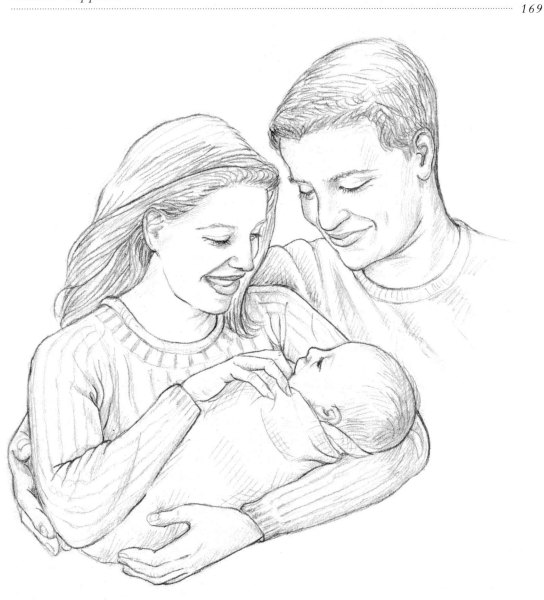

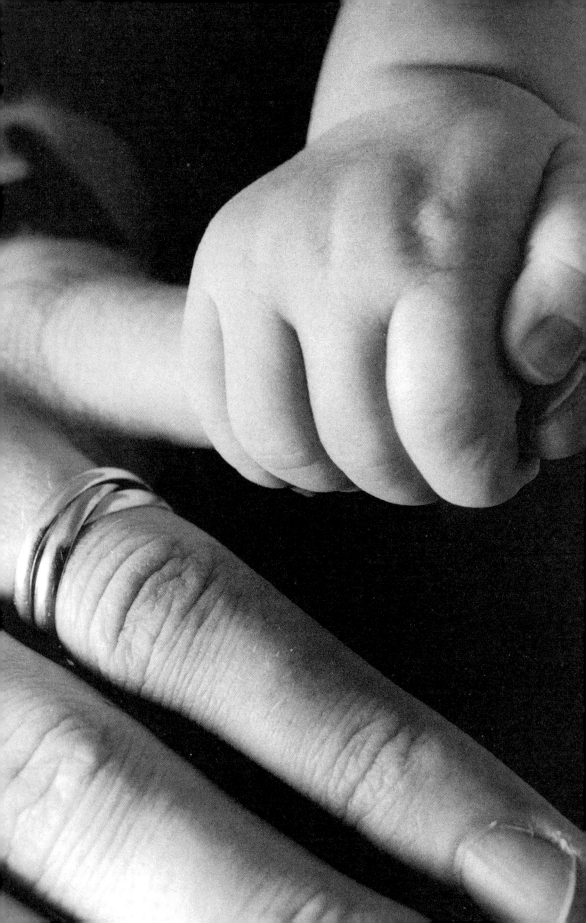

CHAPTER *eight* *Fears and losses*

THERE ARE all sorts of fears and losses involved in becoming pregnant and having a baby. Pregnancy may mean alterations in your daily routine as you cope with tiredness, sickness and clinic appointments. Your old way of looking at the world changes: some things move into sharper focus so that items on the news about people starving, for example, and especially about children suffering are suddenly charged with far stronger emotions than they were before. Pregnancy is a time when women are often excited and optimistic, but it's also a time of anxiety about whether the baby will be healthy, what labour will be like and how they will cope afterwards. As the months pass by, most women become increasingly and sometimes sadly aware that the freedom which they once enjoyed as a single person or as a couple will disappear when the baby is born. During labour, the birth plans they had made when they were pregnant are replaced by the actuality of what happens. When the baby is born, the fantasy baby of pregnancy changes into a real baby with a distinctive appearance and distinctive behaviour. Postnatally, their image of themselves as firm-bodied women who have not borne children is replaced by a body-image which includes a rounded tummy and larger and softer breasts.

FEARS ABOUT NOT COPING WITH LABOUR PAIN

ALTHOUGH DOCTORS have developed sophisticated methods of pain relief for use in labour, and some women feel that they should not have to suffer while they are giving birth, a surprisingly large number of women would prefer to manage without having drugs or drips. Labour is seen as a major hurdle in life which, if you can leap it on your own, will give you great satisfaction. Women often feel that the ability to give birth without medical assistance says something about their strength as a woman. This strong sense of wanting to use your own resources to cope with pain in labour often runs alongside a fear of disappointment should that not be possible, as these three women suggest:

'I shall give it as good a go as I can and then if I feel I need some help, I'll ask for it. If I don't do it myself, I hope I won't feel I've failed.'

'The important thing is not to feel you've failed – but if things go wrong, how can you be sure you won't feel that way?'

'I'm frightened I'm going to give in and ask for an epidural. I really don't want to have an epidural.'

THE LOSS OF THE LABOUR YOU WANTED

BECAUSE THERE is no blueprint for labour, it's impossible to predict what will happen; how a woman copes with pain in labour depends on so many things – how well supported she is by her labour companion and midwife; her personal pain threshold; the environment in which she is giving birth; what position her baby is in inside her; how long the labour is; whether there are any complications . . . and so on. Whatever happens, the woman will inevitably have very definite feelings about her labour after it is over because giving birth is the kind of life experience that you remember for ever:

'The first labour was glorious, idyllic, everything you can dream of and I felt wonderful, but I had a lot of disappointment with the birth of my second baby. The labour was half the length of the first, but very painful and I felt so tired for days afterwards. I felt disappointed not to feel as ecstatic as I had first time round. The second time, the baby was posterior and he was squashed and he came out angry. I was disappointed at the pain and not being able to cope like I coped the first time.'

There may not be much sympathy for a woman who feels low after childbirth because the labour was not as she would have liked it: *'A lot of people say to me, "But you've got a healthy baby, why are you worried? It all turned out all right in the end". But I can't get over how angry and disappointed and mauled I feel because of everything that went wrong in my* labour. I didn't get on with the midwife who was with me and that was a disappointment in itself. I think I could have had a totally different birth if I'd had someone I really trusted.'

Having a caesarean section may be a life-saving measure for both mother and baby, but even when the woman is convinced in her mind that there is a genuine need for her baby to be born this way, her feelings aren't always so logical:

'When I think about loss, I think about my second birth. I had my first baby so positively, at home, a really amazing experience. So I was very shocked when, the second time, I ended up in the middle of the night having an emergency caesarean. There was a hard band on one side of my cervix caused by laser surgery which I'd had between the two babies, and I couldn't dilate beyond 2 cms. I felt I'd been robbed of my birth. The thought that I might never be able to have a vaginal birth again really upsets me.'

Not knowing exactly what happened during the labour can cause women to feel unhappy about their births for years to come: 'I have definite lows about the caesarean and I have "I don't care" phases. At the moment, I'm debating whether or not the caesarean was necessary as I've just been finding out more information. I keep thinking, "If only they'd left me another ten minutes . . . if only . . ." Jo's two and a half now and the disappointment still comes in phases.'

The loss of control which, for some women, sums up their experience of labour either because they feel that they were overwhelmed by pain and didn't behave as they would have liked, or because events meant that they needed a large number of medical interventions to ensure a safe outcome, can be deeply felt: 'You feel cheated that it hasn't all gone the right way, the way that you planned it.'

MEETING A DIFFERENT BABY

IT'S INTRIGUING to imagine while you are pregnant what your baby is going to look like. The moment when a woman sees her baby for the first time and the thoughts she has at that instant are destined to become a very important part of her life experience. It is not uncom-

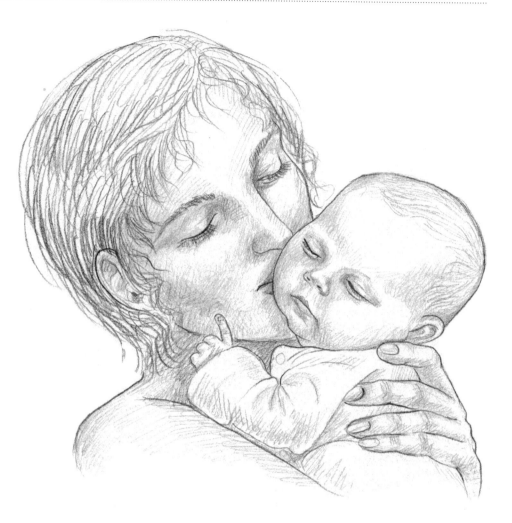

mon for pregnant women to anticipate very vividly that moment of meeting: *'I used to dream that he came out in the night and we had a look at him and he wasn't quite ready so we put him back! And I had that dream a couple of times because I wanted to know what he looked like.'*

'You can have very funny dreams where the baby has your face or your husband's face or an animal's face sometimes!'

When the new baby finally arrives, he or she may look nothing like the media image which we all have of the perfect, clean and smiling baby or the image you had created in your mind's eye:

'I turned over to look at her and saw the fattest baby I had ever seen. She looked like a cross between a pekinese puppy and a Sumo wrestler.'

'Who was this blueish, squinting, skinny thing?'

'I remember looking down and thinking, "Oh my God, it's got purple skin and green hair." I was so shocked. Obviously he'd had his bowels open as he was being born so the sludge had got all over him, and he had a lot of hair and he came out with green hair!'

The baby may not be the sex which the mother had wanted. Women often find it difficult to express their disappointment about this because in many societies, it is unacceptable to grieve over a baby who is perfectly well but simply not of the desired sex:

'I really wanted a girl the third time round because I already had two boys and I was very disappointed to have another boy. I shan't have any more children so I'll never have a little girl now.'

NOT MEETING THE BABY

SOME WOMEN who have had long and very exhausting labours are in no position to greet their babies when they are born and welcome them into the world: *'I can vaguely remember trying to hold the slippery bundle and unravel the cord that was round her. I can't remember what she looked like and that makes me really sad. They took her away and I collapsed back onto some cushions. I didn't even think about where the baby was.'*

The emotions which are experienced at birth may not be what the woman had anticipated: *'Every mum would like to feel this over-whelming love when she first meets her baby, but it doesn't always work that way. I felt nothing for my baby – just vaguely anxious because she looked so blue. I said, "Give her to my husband".'*

A mother who is giving birth to twins may find that her attention is so caught up with what is happening to the baby who has been born first that she misses the moment when the second is born: *'Alarmingly, she didn't cry and she was purple – she was whisked away to the resuscitation trolley. I forgot about the other twin completely because I was so worried about Corrie and our little boy was born with me quite oblivious to him.'*

Mothers whose babies are poorly may also miss the excitement and joy of seeing and holding their babies as soon as they are born: *'I had her at five past nine in the morning and I didn't wake up until eleven when they said, "It's a girl and she's all right". But I was that drugged up, I couldn't go to see her. I kept saying, "Can I go to see her yet, can I go and see her yet?" and they wouldn't let me. They did take a photograph of her which helped and Simon kept rushing off to Special Care, but it was very hard not being able to see her for over 12 hours.'*

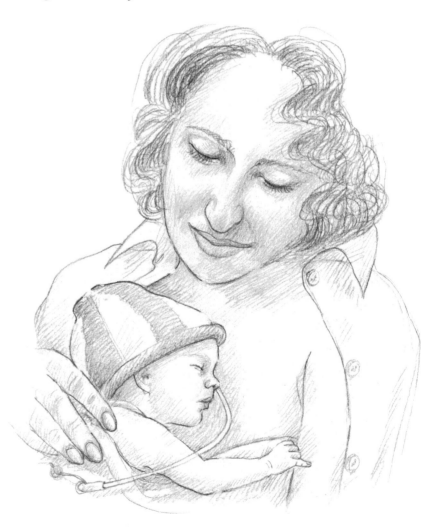

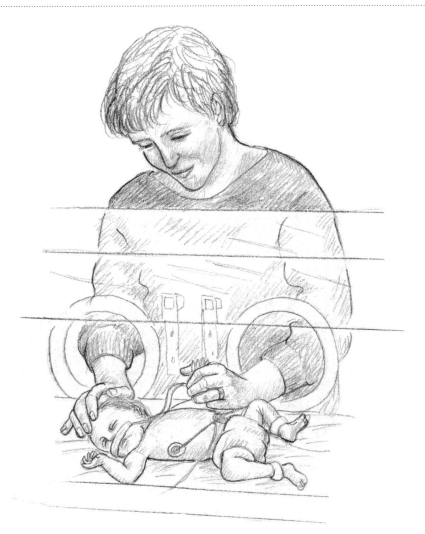

'*She had blue eyes, although she was very grey-looking. I held her for a moment and the eyes were really striking and then she was rushed off to Special Care. I kept thinking, "I want to see my baby; where's my baby gone?" I felt that precious hours were being lost when I should have been with my baby.*'

The shock when you have been expecting to have a gorgeous healthy baby and the reality turns out to be a very small, very sick one is unimaginable: '*Because I am a big person, I envisaged I was going to have this whopping great big baby and when I had this tiny baby that was being tube-fed and I couldn't hold him, and I didn't see him on the day I had him . . . I can't explain what it did to me.*'

A sick baby or two sick babies mean that the mother and her partner have instantly to replace their image of healthy newborns with a very different image. Poorly babies can seem like complete strangers to their parents: *'My partner and I were taken to see the twins in the Special Care Baby Unit. We touched their tiny hands and cried because they were so small. Then we went back to the ward. We felt as if we didn't know our babies at all.'*

Women who go to hospital in order to give birth to their babies eagerly look forward to the day when they will proudly bring their babies home to meet their families, but mothers whose babies need long-term special care have to come home on their own: *'I was OK while I was in hospital, but when I came home and he was still in there, that was hard. When I used to come home after the last visit of the day, I'd cry my eyes out all night because I had to leave him there until the next day.'*

THE DEATH OF A BABY

WHEN BIRTH and death occur close together, and an event which had been anticipated as bringing with it immense happiness turns into a tragedy, parents suffer an emotional free fall unimaginable in its intensity:

'The baby was very still and there was no sound.'

'My baby was discovered to be dead at 38 weeks despite the fact that her heartbeat had been heard quite clearly at 37 weeks. We decided to go home and come back in to induce the baby the following day. When she was born, the midwife took her straight out of the room because we had decided we didn't want to see her; then she came and asked if we were sure about that and we said we would like to see her after all. As soon as we looked at her, we called her Sarah. We knew then that we had lost a member of our family.'

Soon after the first shock comes the rush of questions: *'Why us? Why did it have to happen? What had I done wrong?'*

Hospitals are, in general, far better at looking after grieving parents than they used to be. Parents are given time to hold their baby for as long as they want because if they don't meet their baby, it's very hard to grieve for a person they have never known. When the mother dresses her dead baby in his own clothes and cuddles him and weeps over him, she is acknowledging that this baby was a real little person who was alive and is now dead. Parents are encouraged to take photographs of their baby and can be given a hand or footprint and a lock of the baby's hair. Most hospitals now have a special Book of Remembrance in which parents can write the name of their miscarried or stillborn baby and a few words about him. Some parents find that they cannot do this immediately, but return to the hospital, perhaps many months later, to put their baby's name in the book.

During the initial period of numbness, funeral arrangements have to be made and friends and relatives rally round. But once the funeral is over, bereaved parents can become very isolated. People in general find it difficult to cope with the death of a baby and don't know what to say to the parents. The result is that they sometimes make extremely insensitive comments simply because they are so distressed and embarrassed themselves: *'"You're young; you can have another baby". It was like saying, "Your best friend's died but, don't worry, you can get another one".'*

Nature can also seem very insensitive at this time because, despite the fact that the baby is dead, the mother's breasts still make the milk which would have been needed had he lived: *'For the first three weeks, my sore breasts were a continual reminder of our loss.'*

After the initial period of intense grieving is over, parents often find that what they most need is to talk endlessly about their feelings and their baby:

'Talk, talk, talk is the best therapy.'

'I was very lucky in that a number of friends let me talk about Jo-jo and didn't get embarrassed if I cried. Sometimes they cried too. Talking was my best prescription.'

Women may need to talk to their GP or midwife about their pregnancy to find out why things went wrong. While generally being able to reassure a mother that nothing she did or did not do had any effect on the outcome of her pregnancy, health professionals are still often unable to explain to her why her baby died. It is nonetheless very important to the mother and her partner to have this chance to talk to a professional person so that they have the comfort of knowing they are fully informed.

The best people to talk to are those who have also lost a baby and *really* know what you feel like. Their support is invaluable: *'I found it difficult to talk to my mother, to close family, because you knew they were suffering as well and I didn't want to distress them any more. I had a friend who lost her baby about six weeks before me, and it helped a great deal talking to her.'*

The hospital or community midwife can give the bereaved parents details of how to contact organisations such as the Stillbirth and Neonatal Death Society whose members have all experienced the loss of a baby themselves and who are willing to listen to and support other parents:

'I had to talk to people who had had a similar tragedy and could understand the terrifying emotions I was going through.'

NOT BEING PREGNANT ANY MORE

DESPITE ALL the discomforts and anxieties of pregnancy, many women thoroughly enjoy those nine months when they are the centre of attention and feel proud and special. And however happy the mother is when her baby is born, she can still feel regretful that she isn't pregnant any more:

'I really felt the loss of my bump when I had the baby. I enjoyed people getting out of my way in Sainsbury's and helping me across the road.'

'I loved my stomach right from the very first moment I knew I was pregnant. I sang to my stomach in the shower; I used to rub it. Not having my bump any more feels very sad.'

'I felt wonderful when I was pregnant. I was never alone. If I was frightened, I used to sit and talk to my bump. It gave me great comfort.'

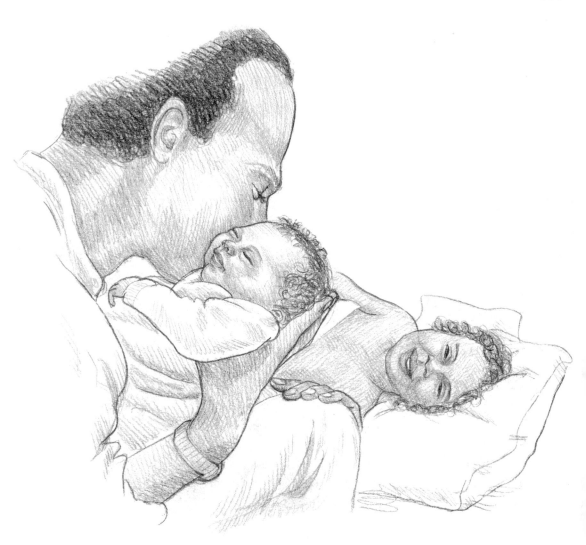

After the birth, people's attention tends to shift away from the woman and onto her baby. For the mother, it's very hard to have carried the baby for nine months, been through labour and then discover that she is apparently less important:

'When you are pregnant, everyone makes a bit of a fuss of you. The minute you have the baby, you come second and you never get the same attention again. The baby's what everyone wants to see; they'll ask you how you are, but it's the baby they're really interested in. It's quite a shock to the system.'

Loss of independence

IT'S HARD to imagine while you are still pregnant just how demanding a new baby can be and how many hours of the day and night are needed to keep up with the feeding and nappy changing and soothing. It could be that we often find becoming a mother very difficult today because we have so many other things that we want to do and are expected to do as well as looking after our babies. There just doesn't seem to be enough time for everything and the sense of frustration when the routine of life which you used to enjoy is turned upside down can be considerable. Women are quite aware when they're pregnant that life will change after the birth of their babies – appreciating just how big that change will be is nearly impossible. *'What I'm frightened of is a loss of energy. I just think I won't have any energy and I might feel poorly and I won't be able to do anything and I'm worried about that. Also I worry about my loss of independence because everyone keeps telling me that my life is never going to be the same again, so I worry about the loss of me as the person I now am.'*

After the baby is born, the freedom which you once enjoyed of being responsible only for yourself is replaced by a burden, which can sometimes seem very heavy, of being entirely responsible for someone else's well-being:

'My baby was so very, very little and I found it overwhelming that he was so dependent on me, really scary.'

'You know that the buck stops with you. You can call your mother and all that, but finally, the buck stops with you. That's very frightening.'

The responsibility can feel all the heavier when the mother is extremely tired. The loss of undisturbed nights and peaceful sleep is a very real one: *'I miss my sleep; that's a real sense of loss.'*

GETTING HELP

IT'S QUITE normal to have a sense of loss as well as happiness after your baby is born. Settling into a new role as a mother requires time and just as your body takes some weeks to recover from labour, so your emotions will take at least as long and probably much longer to calm down. It is often very helpful to be able to talk about your labour and how you feel about your new baby to someone else who will be sympathetic and listen well. Some women find it helpful to write down their birth experiences and keep a diary of the first weeks of motherhood; putting their feelings on paper helps them to understand them: *'I wrote it all down and it made sense. I think it's one of the things that helped me.'*

Some hospitals ensure that every woman has a chance to debrief her labour while she is on the postnatal ward; if you have your baby at home, your midwife may give you the opportunity to talk about what happened when she visits you postnatally. It is very helpful to be able to go over the events of your labour with the midwife who cared for you when your baby was born so that she can explain to you why things happened as they did and ensure that you have no unanswered questions which might cause you concern in the future. Many women feel that: *'Every hospital should run a debriefing service, otherwise we carry these experiences around for ever.'*

The best form of ongoing support after you become a mother is likely to be other women who are also mothers. Seeking them out if your circle of friends doesn't include women with babies may take some effort, but it's crucial. Other mothers of tiny babies *know* how you are feeling, and are quite definitely the people most able to offer you sound, practical advice and support.

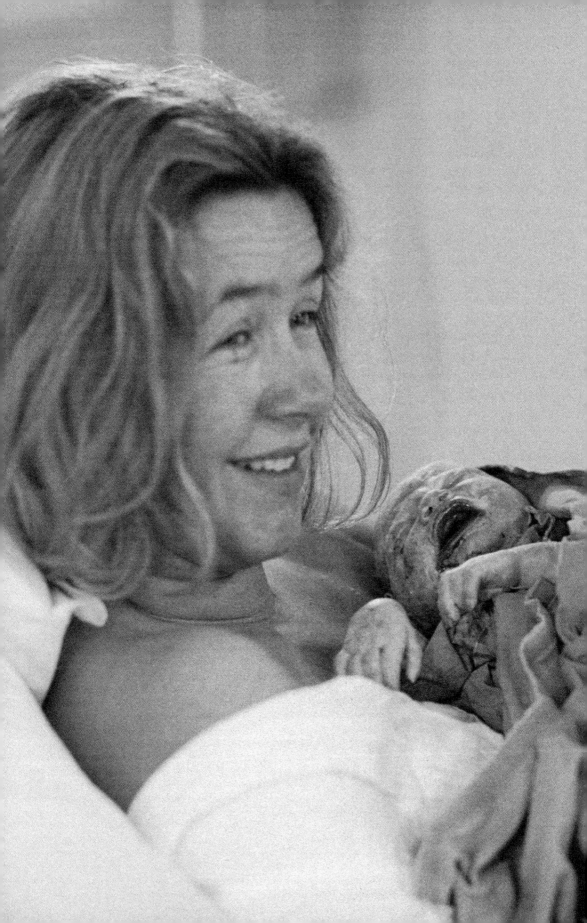

CHAPTER *nine* The
first days

THE FIRST few hours and days after the birth of your baby are filled with a huge variety of experiences – both physical and emotional. Your body is suddenly no longer pregnant; it is undergoing tremendous changes as the uterus shrinks in size and starts to return to its pre-pregnancy state. All the fluid which accumulated in your body while you were pregnant has to be got rid of and many women who have just given birth often find that they need to go to the toilet as frequently as they did at the end of their pregnancies. The breasts are responding to hormones which instruct them to make first colostrum and then mature milk; if you decide not to breastfeed your baby, the breasts have to respond to the fact that the baby is not being put to the breast and no milk is required. Coupled with all this frantic physiological activity inside you is the mental exhaustion which many women feel after labour, if not immediately, then a few days later.

The reaction of friends and family to the announcement that the baby has been safely born is naturally one of delight: the news is 'absolutely wonderful' and the parents should feel 'over the moon'. Mothers themselves often find that their emotions are turbulent during the first days after the birth and they have times of being extremely happy and times of being extremely unhappy. A joyous birth may turn into a bout of crying and despair when the baby blues set in a few days later. Women can find themselves trying to keep up an appearance of being the delighted and caring mother while feeling very insecure, very aware of the heavy responsibility of the baby and resentful of the loss of personal space which they are now experiencing.

EXAMINING YOUR BABY AT BIRTH

The Midwife's Check

Within the first hour of his birth, the midwife will examine your baby carefully to make sure that he is healthy. She will check:

- His eyes: to see if they are a normal distance apart and that each lens is clear
- His mouth: to make sure that the hard palate is complete and not cleft and that the baby has no teeth. (Very occasionally, a baby is born with a couple of teeth which are generally loose and need taking out in case the baby breathes them into his lungs.)
- His breathing: to see that he is breathing through his nose and not through his mouth
- His head: to assess the shape of the skull and check that the soft spots on the baby's head are normal
- His chest and abdomen: to check that the breathing movements of the baby's chest are regular and that his abdomen is round
- The stump of the umbilical cord: to check that there are three blood vessels. (The midwife will probably remove the metal forceps which were clipped onto the cord when your baby was born and replace them with a plastic clamp.)
- The genitals: to ensure that the penis is open at the end, or that a girl baby has two openings, one from her vagina and one from her urethra
- The back passage: to make sure that it is open. (The midwife will take the baby's temperature by putting a thermometer gently into his back passage; this is the most accurate way of finding a baby's temperature.)
- His hands and feet: to make sure there are ten fingers and ten toes! and that the baby can move his wrists and ankles normally
- His spine: to make sure the backbone has formed properly.

The midwife will measure the circumference around the baby's head and usually his length from the top of his head to his heels; she will also weigh him.

The Paediatrician's Check

Your baby will be examined during the first few days of his life by a paediatrician who will:

- Listen to your baby's heart and lungs
- Feel your baby's abdomen to check whether the organs inside seem the normal size
- Check your baby's reflexes to make sure that his nervous system has developed properly
- Test your baby's hips. This is a very important test. Some babies have what is described as 'clicky hips' because the sockets in the hip bone which hold the long bones of his legs firmly in place are too shallow and allow the bones to slip out. If the baby is not treated for this condition, he will have great difficulty in crawling and walking. Fortunately, if clicky hips are noticed soon after the baby's birth, they can be treated so that the sockets of the hips deepen and keep the long bones in place. The treatment involves putting the baby in double nappies to keep his legs wide apart, or using a plastic 'frog splint' over his nappy which is also designed to hold his legs apart. The baby needs to wear double nappies or the splint for several weeks. In most cases, the problem is then solved. A very few babies go on to need an operation when they are one or two years old.

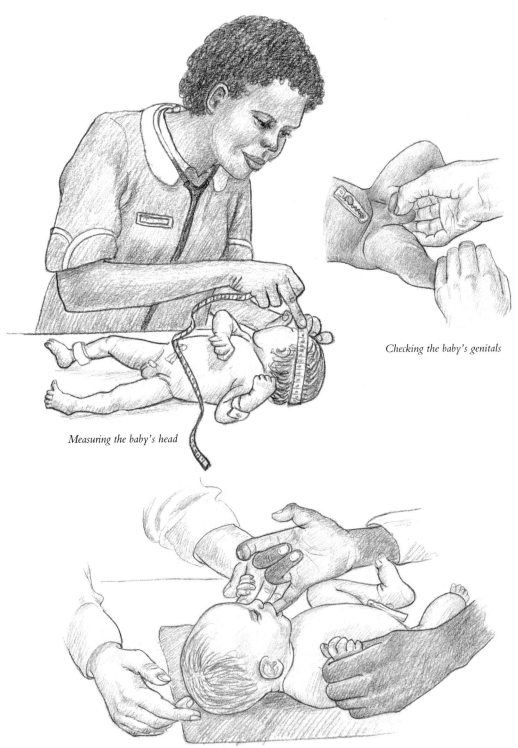

Measuring the baby's head

Checking the baby's genitals

Checking the baby's palate

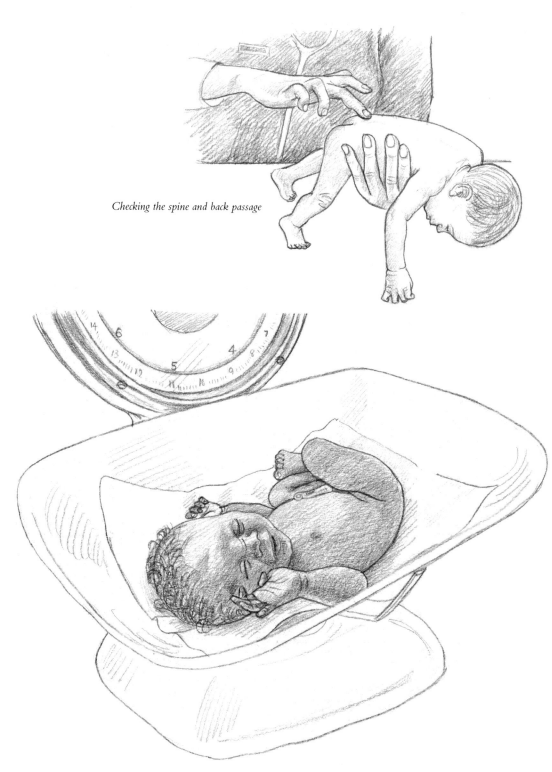

Checking the spine and back passage

THE FIRST TWENTY-FOUR HOURS

WOMEN REACT in very different ways during the immediate aftermath of labour. Some feel exhausted and want only to sleep; others are very alert and quite unable to sleep:

'When I had him, I couldn't sleep for the first night at all. I was awake most of the night just looking at him and his face was towards me and I couldn't quite believe what had happened.'

'I felt calm and had lots of sleep.'

Both types of reactions are entirely normal. Simply wanting to be left alone and to go to sleep after your labour is over does not make you a bad mother. If, on the other hand, you can't sleep and want to spend all your time looking at your baby, that's fine as well. Some babies seem to want the reassurance of feeding frequently in the first twenty-four hours after birth; others are too busy looking at the new world they find themselves in and too excited to feed.

'The baby slept all night – she's never done it since.'

'She didn't sleep very much during the first day; I think she was as excited as I was.'

'Tom didn't feed much during the first twenty-four hours. I felt like he was recovering and he was allowing me time to recover, and he didn't really wake me very much.'

'He fed a lot during the first twenty-four hours.'

THE APGAR SCORE

(named after Dr Virginia Apgar)

After your baby has been born and given to you to hold, the midwife will make a quick assessment of how healthy he is. She does this by noting his:

- Colour
- Heart rate
- Breathing
- Movements
- Reflexes

and giving him a score of 0, 1 or 2 for each of these things. Your baby is given an APGAR score one minute after his birth and five minutes after. Typically, he might have a score of 7 at one minute and then as his breathing becomes stronger and his colour changes from bluey-purple to pink, a score of 10 at five minutes. If the Apgar score is low at one minute and especially if it is low at five minutes, the midwife will call a doctor to look at your baby and see whether he needs some special help.

YOUR BABY'S FIRST FEED

If you want to breastfeed your baby, it's helpful if you try putting him to the breast as soon as he is born. Newborn babies are generally very alert, and they remain wide awake for quite a few hours. You can make the most of this period while he is so interested in the world to start learning with him about breastfeeding.

The most important thing to get right is the position of your baby on the breast – ask your midwife to help you. If you make sure he takes your breast properly right from the beginning, *you* will avoid getting sore nipples and *he* is likely to be a much more contented baby who can fill his stomach easily.

Don't worry if your baby doesn't seem to feed very much, or doesn't appear to get the hang of breastfeeding at all! There's plenty of time for you both to learn. Babies don't need many feeds in the first twenty-four hours of their lives; they often spend much of them sleeping and some will only want to go to the breast two or three times in the day. That's quite normal, although it's also quite normal if your baby wants to feed much more frequently.

The first kind of milk which your baby receives from you is colostrum. Colostrum contains antibodies to all sorts of diseases and will give your baby a marvellous start in life, but there isn't much of it. Don't worry: your baby will certainly not starve while he waits for you to make more milk. Nature has made sure that he has built up plenty of stores of fat during the final weeks in your uterus, and these will keep him going until your mature milk starts to come through after a few days.

Remember that breastfed babies don't need anything except breast milk. They don't need water and they don't need formula milk. They just need you!

Newborn babies need very little milk in the first day of life and if your baby goes to the breast only a couple of times or has only two or three bottles, there's no need to worry.

HOW LONG TO STAY IN HOSPITAL

SOME WOMEN find it reassuring to spend several days in hospital after the birth; it feels very secure to know that there is always a midwife or doctor to hand if there is a problem with the baby. Others find the environment of the hospital stressful and their choice is to go home as quickly as possible: *'I went home 20 hours after I'd had the baby. I didn't want to stay in any longer. The staff that were trying to help me breastfeed were always touching, always interfering. Conflicting advice from everybody.'*

Conflicting advice is less likely if the woman is cared for by a midwife or a couple of midwives whom she knows already: *'During 36 hours in hospital, I must have had four different midwives show me how to feed the baby.'*

THE SUPPORT which the woman receives during the first days and weeks with her new baby is vital. If she is in hospital after the birth, the attitude of staff can make all the difference between her feeling strong enough to cope with a completely new life-style and feeling totally inadequate:

BABIES WHO NEED SPECIAL CARE

Some babies need to be cared for in the Special Care Baby Unit (SCBU) or in the Neonatal Intensive Care Unit (NNICU) after they are born. Babies may need special care when:

- They have been born prematurely, that is, before 37 weeks of pregnancy
- They are very small even if they have been in the uterus for more than 37 weeks
- They have had a difficult time during labour
- They are twins or triplets or more
- They are born with a problem with a major organ such as heart or kidneys
- They have a disability, such as when they have Down's syndrome
- They are having problems with breathing.

What you can do if your baby is in the Special Care Unit

- Stroke your baby, hold his hand and touch him. If you are allowed to, give him lots of cuddles.

  Babies who are ill at birth may need to have a lot of unpleasant things done to them – they may need to have drips put in their hands or head; they may need a tube passed through their nose down into their tummy; they may need to have blood samples taken; they may need a tube put into their lungs to help them breathe. However gently done, these things probably hurt the baby and he needs comforting afterwards. Poorly babies have emotional needs as well as physical ones. And so do you! You need

to hold your baby as much as possible and he needs you to hold him.

- Express breast milk for your baby; a midwife will show you how to use a breast pump. Your milk can be given to your baby down a tube if that is how he is being fed. Learn how to tube feed your baby yourself
- Wash your baby and change his nappies
- Ask if it is possible for you to stay in the hospital while your baby is in the Special Care Unit. Some hospitals have accommodation for parents whose babies are poorly
- Talk to the nurses and doctors; ask them to explain your baby's treatment. Ask again if you don't understand anything. Say that you want an honest account of your baby's condition
- When you telephone the Special Care Unit, ask to speak to the midwife who is responsible for the care of your baby
- Take lots of photographs of your baby – most new parents are keen to start an album straight away; there's no reason why you shouldn't, too – you also have a baby
- Put some small toys which you have chosen for your baby in his cot
- When your baby can be dressed, dress him in the clothes you have bought for him. Even if they're much too big, they're his, and wearing them will help you to see him as *your* baby rather than the hospital's
- Ask for help at home – from your mother, mother-in-law, sister, relatives, friends – anyone who will simply help you cope without making any demands on you.

'One day, the midwife told me off for carrying my baby. She told me to wheel him around. I was not to carry this baby and that really upset me. I didn't know what was the right thing to do.'

EXPRESSING BREAST MILK FOR YOUR BABY IN SPECIAL CARE

An electric breast pump is certainly the most efficient way of expressing milk. You will be able to use a pump at the hospital while you are there and you may be able to borrow one to take home if you are discharged from the hospital before your baby is. If you can't borrow a pump from the hospital, you should be able to hire one from either:

The National Childbirth Trust
or
La Leche League

- With an electric pump, you can pump both breasts at the same time and this will help build up your milk supply as quickly as possible

- Expect to pump very little milk to begin with; the quantity you collect will gradually increase if you pump regularly

- Take advice from the midwives in the Special Care Unit about how often to pump and for how long

- Your expressed milk can be fed to your baby through the tube in his nose. When he becomes stronger, he will no longer accept the tube, but he may still not be ready to be fully breastfed. During this change-over period, you can feed him your expressed milk using a tiny cup specially designed for small or poorly babies. It's better to avoid giving your baby a bottle if you intend to breastfeed because bottle-fed babies feed from a teat in a completely different way from breastfed babies.

'The realisation that this was it – here was the baby with me for the rest of my life – hit me hard the first couple of days. But the support I had from the hospital was very good; the midwives were brilliant – very patient.'

While some women thoroughly enjoy being with other new mothers on the postnatal ward and find their company very supportive, others long for the privacy of their own homes: *'I was glad to be at home, especially with stitches and everything. It was nice to be in my own bathroom.'*

Being with other women on a postnatal ward may not be supportive if you are the only one bottle-feeding or the only one breastfeeding: *'Everyone else had their bottles. I couldn't relax. Every time I breastfed, somebody pulled the curtains around me.'*

Recent media stories about babies being snatched from hospitals may also influence some women to take their babies to the safety of their own homes as soon as possible: *'While I was in hospital, I used to sleep with the baby in bed with me and I was worried all the time in case she was stolen.'*

In the end, how long a woman wants to stay on the postnatal ward should be her own decision. Women who are initially very nervous about their new responsibilities and highly dependent on professional staff will, as long as they are not rushed, gradually grow in confidence until they are ready and happy to go home: *'I stayed in hospital five days. The first couple of days I didn't want to go home because I thought I would never cope. By the end I was ready to go home, happy to go home.'*

BRINGING YOUR BABY HOME

EVEN WHEN the woman has made her own decision that now is the right time to go home, leaving the hospital requires a lot of courage: *'I'd been in hospital for a week and I said, "I'm doing fine. I want to go home". But once I was in the car and going home, I felt all panicky because now I was on my own; this was it.'*

Often, the person who gives the reassurance which the mother needs is her baby: *'I was terrified about leaving hospital. I thought, "There are so many things I don't know how to do; I don't know how to breastfeed properly", and I was convinced that some major disaster would happen as soon as I got home. What helped was that the baby had a really good feed just after I got back and I started to think, "Maybe it's all right".'*

The natural anxiety which women feel about bringing the baby out of hospital is often balanced by immense pride and excitement. The

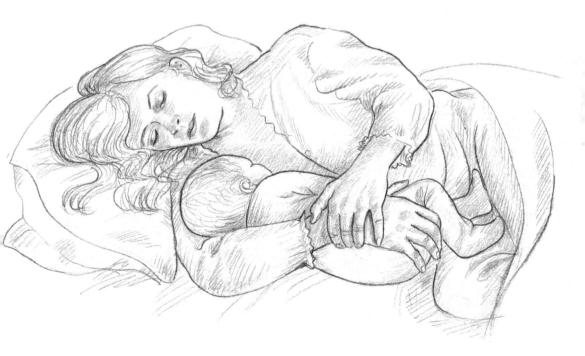

house takes on a new dimension because now it is home for one more person than it was before:

'_I remember taking her on a tour when we got home, showing her the kitchen and showing her her bedroom and it was just lovely._'

'_The first night at home, I just lay there and I felt so excited, just feeling sick with excitement because it was something so new and so lovely._'

ONCE THE front door shuts, however, and you find yourself completely independent from health professionals (until your midwife's first visit), small worries can become enormous ones:

'_I never knew babies could make so much noise at night. Babies grunt when they breathe and that really worried me._'

'_He slept quite well on the first night home and would have slept better if I hadn't constantly been poking him just to make sure he was still breathing._'

This kind of extreme anxiety is absolutely typical of the first days of parenthood and there's probably no way of avoiding it. It's a natural process which ensures that babies are very well cared for when they are at their most vulnerable and just getting started in life. The constant reassurance which new mothers need means that they ask for help and information from others more experienced than themselves. This is one of the ways in which they are able to grow in knowledge about babycare and confidence in themselves as mothers:

'_I was in a panic about how hot he was. I got out this booklet about cot death and I rang my mother and said, "I don't know how hot he's meant to be." I was in a real panic. She calmed me down._'

COPING WITH VISITORS

SOME WOMEN love being at the centre of attention when they come home from hospital; they feel on top of the world, have no worries about coping and enjoy showing off their baby to as many people as possible: '_I just found it all exhilarating. There were people phoning up all_

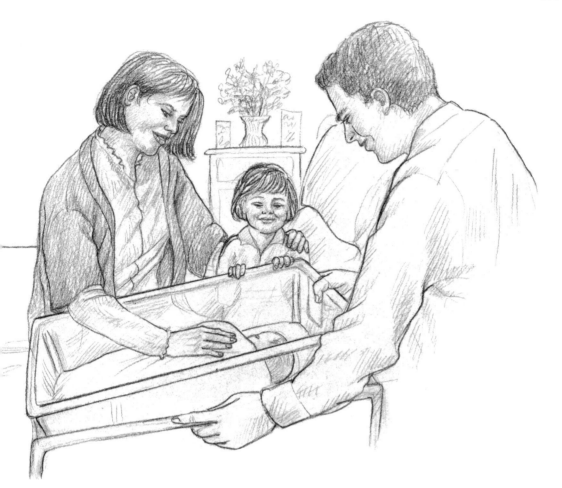

the time and loads of visitors and I found it was just like one long party. We saw everybody that we know and I really enjoyed that. I didn't find it intrusive. It helped me to get back to normal.'

Others, however, feel that they are still recovering from the birth and need time to be quiet and get used to being a new family: *'I just wanted the three of us – together.'*

Having people try to help you is not always a blessing. Help in the early days frequently comes from those nearest to you: your partner, your own mother and father and your in-laws. All these people are busy adjusting to their new roles as a father or as grandparents just as you are adjusting to being a mother. They may feel unsure about

TESTS YOUR BABY WILL HAVE IN THE FIRST DAYS OF LIFE

Guthrie Test

Four or five days after your baby's birth, the midwife will ask to take a few drops of blood from his heel. It is likely that you will find this a much more painful experience than your baby does although he will probably cry inconsolably – but it is worth while. Your baby's blood is tested for the following conditions:

- Phenylketonuria – the baby cannot break down the protein in his food properly; the half-way broken-down products are poisonous and accumulate in the brain causing mental disability
- Galactosaemia – the baby cannot digest sugar properly and may have problems with his sight, his liver, kidneys and brain
- Hypothyroidism – this is the medical term for having too little thyroid hormone; the baby will become seriously mentally disabled.

The important thing to understand about these conditions is that they do not mean the baby is mentally disabled at birth, but only that he will become so if he is not treated. The Guthrie Test enables health professionals to diagnose that the baby has one of these conditions and to start treating him as soon as possible. A baby treated for phenylketonuria or galactosaemia or hypothyroidism from the early days of his life will thrive and become a normally intelligent adult.

Blood Tests for Jaundice

A day or so after their births, some babies become rather yellow in appearance almost as if they have a suntan, and this means that they have jaundice. It is quite usual for babies to become slightly jaundiced. Whilst they are in the uterus, they have a large number of red blood cells to carry oxygen around their bodies; after they are born, they don't need as many red blood cells and start to break some of them down. The broken-down red blood cells are passed out in the baby's urine, but if this doesn't happen quickly enough, they remain in the body and stain the skin yellow. In most cases, the best way of getting rid of jaundice is to feed your baby as often as you can. Breastfed babies don't need to be given bottles to increase their intake of milk; they just need to be put to the breast more frequently.

By the seventh day of the baby's life, the jaundice has nearly always gone. A few babies have severe jaundice and they will have their blood tested to see if they need phototherapy to help them. This means laying the baby, naked, except for a bandage to protect his eyes, underneath a blue light. It is hard for mothers whose babies need phototherapy because they are separated from their babies in the very early days just when cuddling them feels so important. However, phototherapy is generally only given for a day or two, and you can, of course, take your baby out from under the light and hold him while you are feeding him.

what to do and what not to do for you and anxious about offending if they handle the baby in a way which you don't like. Some people are instinctively good at helping and get on with things without making a fuss or making you feel obliged to them. Others end up creat-

VITAMIN K

Vitamin K is needed in order to make your blood clot properly. Newborn babies have very little and a small number suffer from bleeding problems in the first few days or weeks of their lives. To protect these few, it has become customary to give vitamin K to all babies at birth. In the past, it was generally given by injection.

You may have noticed that vitamin K has been in the news recently. This is because research carried out in the UK found that babies who were given an injection of vitamin K at birth were more at risk of developing cancer in childhood than babies who were not given vitamin K or who had it given to them by mouth.

Since this research was done, more studies have been carried out which have found *no link* between giving babies injections of vitamin K and their getting cancer later on in life.

It is now difficult to know what it is best to do. At the moment, the Department of Health has issued no guidelines for vitamin K although the British Paediatric Association recommends giving it to babies by mouth. Each hospital has drawn up its own rules.

- Some continue to give vitamin K by injection to every newborn baby unless the parents object
- Some give vitamin K by mouth to all newborn babies (the trouble with this is that there is no preparation of vitamin K which is made to be given by mouth; what the babies get is the solution of vitamin K normally given by injection)
- Some give vitamin K by mouth to all newborn babies and one or two further doses to babies who are breastfed.

Breastfed babies have particularly low levels of vitamin K. Nobody knows why. Although this apparently puts them at greater risk of having a bleeding problem, it may be that their low level of vitamin K protects them from something else which we don't yet know about.

So you need to ask about the policy regarding vitamin K at the hospital where you are going to give birth. Or, if you are having your baby at home, ask your midwife which routine she generally follows. If you want to make your own decision about vitamin K, discuss it with your GP, midwife or consultant preferably before your baby is born.

ing more work than there was originally: *'When I arrived home, I had my mother-in-law there. I could have done without that to be quite honest. I just felt so tired and I would have liked time to unpack my bag and have a wash and things like that. I felt very tired and I was making tea and I was thinking, "Well, this isn't right!" I was glad when she went.'*

The best kind of support comes from someone who will simply get on with the household tasks and let you get on with the baby: *'My mother-in-law came over from Australia, otherwise I wouldn't have coped. She made sure the laundry basket wasn't overflowing, cleaned the toilet, and*

POSTNATAL EXERCISE AND DISCUSSION CLASSES

Postnatal exercise classes are becoming very popular and are carefully designed to ensure that you get your body back into shape without overstretching yourself. Classes are run by:

- Hospital physiotherapy departments
- Y.M.C.A.
- Leisure centres – their postnatal exercise classes often include a free swim afterwards
- The National Childbirth Trust – the Trust trains its own postnatal exercise teachers and runs six-week courses in many areas. Your local teacher may also be trained as a discussion leader and after you have exercised, you will have the chance to enjoy a cup of coffee with the other mothers on the course and talk through any problems you might be having.

You will probably have to pay a fee for these classes, but if you can't afford it, say so and you will almost certainly be able to get a discount.

insisted that I ate. She made endless, endless cups of tea. I did nothing except look after the baby.'

It is probably more common than it was a generation ago for partners to get involved in babycare; some men are extremely keen to shoulder their share of the day-to-day routines as early as possible: *'My boyfriend couldn't stop bathing Ricardo. Every time he had a pooey nappy, he'd say, "Oh, he'd better have a bath", and he'd put him in the bath and I just let him get on with it because that was what he enjoyed doing.'*

Being able to accept help from your partner means that you have time for yourself, and watching him playing with the baby can be very special: *'I think men were deprived really until quite recently but it's much easier for them now just to be with their babies. It's really nice to watch Joss and Lisa together, apart from giving me a break!'*

Other women find it very difficult indeed to let their partners have a go at looking after the baby and learn by making their own mistakes: *'Julian was very good; he used to take Oliver away when he was crying in the night, but I used to get really wound up about the way he was looking after him as it wasn't exactly the way I wanted him to do it. It was stupid really that I got so tense when all he was doing was trying to relieve me of worry.'*

'I was really poorly and I remember feeling absolutely panic-stricken when I thought my husband was going to look after Anjali.'

Keeping in touch with each other's feelings by talking to each other and, if at all possible, having time together away from the baby can help to resolve difficulties. When a couple can work together as a team, the responsibility of caring for a new baby certainly seems much lighter: *'I wasn't worried; I felt that I could cope – Martin and I did things together.'*

RECOVERING PHYSICALLY FROM THE BIRTH

IN OUR SOCIETY, women do not expect to be poorly after giving birth to a baby. They expect to take labour in their stride and to be back to normal very quickly. However, even a usually strong and healthy woman can feel very shaky after she has had a baby and it's important to give yourself enough time to recover properly: *'I can remember being taken aback by how long it took me to recover physically after the labour. On the second night, the baby wouldn't settle for two or three hours and I was trying to carry him around with my legs feeling like jelly and I was shocked by how weak I was.'*

'The staircase looked like a mountain and I had to rest every two or three steps and then I crawled along the corridor to the bedroom.'

Recovering from a caesarean section generally takes quite a long time although some mothers are up and about surprisingly quickly: *'I was given very good pain relief in hospital and came home after six days. My scar was fully healed within a week of the birth and I have not had any pain since leaving hospital. In fact, it's hard to believe I had major abdominal surgery.'*

Other women take much longer to recover than this; it's not a question of strength of personality, it's just that each person's response to surgery is different:

'The first time you sit up after a section, it feels like fire. You have to haul yourself up with your arms. And when you first have to stand up, you cannot stand straight because of your wound, and you tend to bend over to prevent the scar from pulling. It took me at least six weeks before I felt normal again and about nine months before the final twinges of pain from the scar disappeared.'

It's very important for a woman who has had a caesarean to have some help when she gets home; local councils used always to provide

YOUR BODY AFTER YOUR BABY IS BORN

After your baby is born, your body has to get back to how it was before you became pregnant. There are a number of things which you can do in the first few days after giving birth which will help this process along.

- *Get up and about* as soon as you are able. This will help you in all sorts of ways:
  - You feel better psychologically if you're not lying in bed all the time
  - You prevent blood pooling in your legs which will make you prone to varicose veins and, more seriously, to getting clots in your veins
  - You help your uterus to empty properly. After giving birth, you will have a heavy discharge, like a period, which is called the lochia and changes from red, to pink to creamy brown over the course of two or three weeks. You may also find that you pass some clots of blood in the first days after the birth; this is normal although your midwife will want to know what they were like and, if possible, you should show them to her
  - You can pass urine more easily. Some women find it difficult to wee after they've had a baby because their bladder has been bruised during the birth. It's much easier to have a wee on the toilet in private than perched on a bedpan in bed!

- Have a *good diet* – lots of women are slightly or very anaemic after giving birth. You can help get your strength back if you choose to eat foods rich in iron such as green leafy vegetables and red meat. Vitamin C helps your body absorb the iron in your diet, so plenty of fresh fruit is also a good idea. Choose foods that are rich in fibre to help your bowels – potatoes with their jackets on, wholemeal bread, bran-based cereals and unpeeled fruit

- Do your *pelvic floor exercises* regularly which means several times a day. If you have stitches in your perineum, the exercises will help you heal more quickly by ensuring a good supply of blood to them

- *Ask for help* – the early days with a new baby can be and often are exhausting. Accept help from anyone who offers. In many cultures, women have no household duties for several weeks after the birth of their babies

- *Rest* – easier said than done! You have to be strict with yourself so that when the baby is asleep, you relax. Don't worry if you can't get to sleep – simply take the telephone off the hook, watch television, have something to eat or close your eyes.

a home-help for every mother who'd had a caesarean – sadly, that's no longer the case. Women now have to find their own carers, but if someone can come to stay with you and relieve you of the day-to-day chores, your recovery is likely to be much quicker.

The changes which happened in your body during the nine months of pregnancy take at least several weeks to be reversed. For example, it's quite normal to have a very heavy loss after giving birth. This is a mixture of blood and mucus and is called the lochia; it is much heavier than a period and generally lasts much longer, on average a couple of weeks: *'Do be prepared for a lot of blood afterwards for the first couple of days; buy disposable pants. It took six weeks for my blood loss to stop completely.'*

If you have had a lot of stitches in your perineum and even if you have only been bruised, it may be a while before you are able to sit down comfortably: *'I was bruised although I didn't have stitches. It was uncomfortable to sit down, although not so bad going to the toilet. If I sat down for long periods and then stood up, the blood rushing to the sore parts certainly was painful!'*

SOME WOMEN find that they get quite severe after-birth pains; these are uncommon with a first baby, but fairly common with subsequent babies. The uterus continues to contract at intervals for a few days after the labour is over. Putting the baby to the breast often stimulates afterpains because the hormone which releases the milk from the breasts also makes the uterus contract:

'Especially second time round, for the first few days I found it was like having period pains every time I put her to the breast. I had noticed it first time round, but it was definitely worse second time.'

Finally, it should be said that some women, although perhaps not many, have no problems *at all* after their babies are born and bounce back to health immediately: *'I just didn't have any problems recovering. I was fitter when I was pregnant with Alexandra than I had ever been before and I think it carried over. I did get very tired about two weeks after she was born, but then I went to stay for a few days with my mum and I was fine. I must admit I was surprised; I thought I would be slopping around for weeks feeling tired and uncomfortable.'*

RECOVERING EMOTIONALLY

NOBODY HAS yet come up with a really good explanation for why so many women have what are called 'the baby blues' a few days after the birth of their babies. It's quite common in maternity hospitals to

FEELING DEPRESSED

Women may feel low in the first weeks and months after having a baby for a variety of very good reasons:

- **Changed life-style** – However determined you were before your baby arrived that he would not prevent you from doing all the things you used to do, you may well find that your life does change radically and that you have to fall in with what your baby wants rather than the other way round.

- **Changes in relationships** – The people who are important to you will see you differently now that you are a mother. Your partner may feel – and you may feel – that you are no longer his friend and lover, but someone whose body and energy have been taken over by the baby.

- **Loneliness** – It's easy to get trapped within the four walls of your home when you have a new baby. Going out can be very complicated: you have to take nappies, wipes, a changing mat, sleepsuits and perhaps bottles. Staying at home may seem much easier, but not seeing anyone for days and not having any adult conversation are almost bound to make you feel low.

- **Tiredness** – Most people become bad tempered and miserable and feel they can't cope with life when they are tired. The vast majority of new mothers are very, very tired during the first weeks and months and sometimes years, of their babies' lives.

GETTING OUT OF THE HOUSE

- Be determined that you *are* going out
- Give yourself plenty of time to get everything ready:
  two spare nappies
  bag to put dirty nappies in
  nappy wipes
  clean sleepsuit
  tissues
  bottle made up with formula if you're bottle-feeding your baby
  breast pads if you're breastfeeding
  your own bag with the things you need
- If possible, try to feed your baby about an hour before you're going out and change her so that she's settled
- Make sure that you've also made time to go to the toilet, brush your hair and put on some make-up if you normally wear it so that you feel confident to meet other people
- Go out!

find a ward full of women crying their hearts out while the midwife explains that they're all three days post-delivery and everyone has got the blues together! It may be a combination of changing levels of hormones, of tiredness and of the growing realisation that life will never be the same again. Often, a very small incident will trigger a flood of tears:

'I woke during the night and I thought, "What if there's a Third World War and we're all blown up in a nuclear explosion. How could I possibly have brought a baby into this world?" And I felt absolutely desperate and I

MEETING OTHER MUMS

Having a baby gives you a wonderful opportunity to make new friends but it demands a certain amount of effort on your part. It is worth it; the friends you make will become your most useful sources of information about *everything* you need to know as a parent:

- Tips for soothing crying babies
- Which shops are the best for baby equipment
- How to amuse a toddler on a wet Sunday afternoon
- Coping with children who are faddy eaters
- How good the local playgroups are etc etc etc . . .

Your local library is an excellent place to get information about where Mother and Baby/Toddler Groups are running in your area. Look for notices in shop windows and at leisure centres. Ask other mums – they will certainly know. Groups are run by:

- Health centres – many now offer six week postnatal courses with a chance to discuss the joys and worries of early parenthood
  Cost: probably free
- Local churches – you don't have to be a church-goer to attend the Mother and Toddler Group
  Cost: about £1 a session
- The National Childbirth Trust – the Trust's Mother and Toddler Groups are often called Open Houses; they may be held in a community centre, or in someone's home
  Cost: between 50p and £1 a session; free in many parts of the country
- Community Centres
  Cost: a small sum or may well be free

Going regularly to the Baby Clinic at your local surgery or health centre is also a good way of getting to know other mums.

---

got through a box and a half of tissues before Peter arrived the next morning.'

'I remember being on the ward by myself and crying, thinking, "I've got a baby and what am I going to do!"'

'I sobbed my heart out sitting by the fridge. Andy offered to go out to do the shopping and I gave him a list and he didn't buy any of the things I wanted and they were all the wrong brands and I didn't have anything I needed and I just sat down with the fridge door open and sobbed. I couldn't help it.'

Your confidence about being a mother will be boosted immeasurably by having people around you who don't offer their own opinions or criticise you, but simply let you get on with caring for your baby in your own way: 'My mother came for a stay when I left hospital and I don't know what I would have done without her. Not that she did very much, but

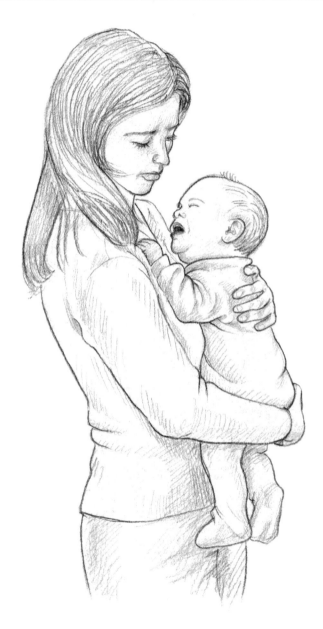

she was a very comforting, reassuring presence for me. She didn't look after the baby; she let me do that and often said what a really good job I was making of it. Her saying that meant a lot.'

The baby blues can last for just a few hours or a few days, but they nearly always pass: *'I was fine until about two days after I came home and then I got very miserable. I went from being high to being miserable, but it didn't last very long, a couple of days.'*

IF YOUR baby blues go on for weeks and weeks, then you are probably suffering from a more serious depression which you need to talk to your doctor or health visitor about. If you can't face seeing a health professional, at least talk to somebody about how you feel. There are excellent treatments and counselling services available now to help women who suffer from postnatal depression.

FEELINGS AFTER A CAESAREAN

RECOVERING emotionally from a caesarean means, for some women, coming to terms both with the fact that their baby wasn't born without intervention, and with an altered body-image. While many mothers feel entirely happy about the decision to have a caesarean and recognise that undergoing major surgery in order to give birth is certainly not an easy option, others are dissatisfied with themselves and feel that not being able to have a vaginal delivery is a failure: *'I had a lot of emotional problems afterwards. I felt like a failure as a mother for not being able to give birth 'properly' and I felt guilty that I had somehow let my partner down for not having the birth that we had planned and discussed.'*

The scar is a constant reminder of the way in which the baby was born, and some women find that their mental unhappiness translates itself into physical weakness, which can take a long time to overcome: *'I hate my tummy – it's like an overhang over the scar. It's really affecting my body image. It has taken me at least a year to get some kind of self-confidence back into me, particularly regarding my physical ability – I used to be very fit and strong but I'm only just beginning to think, "Yes, I can do that".'*

Recovery from emotional trauma requires the support of people who will simply listen to your story, and try to empathise with your feelings, without making any judgements. It's helpful to think about whether you have a friend like this who is good at listening or know of someone who has been through the same experience (both in terms of having a caesarean and in terms of feeling unhappy about it afterwards):

'*The best thing was a friend who'd also had an emergency section coming to talk to me frankly about how I felt.*'

'*For me, coming to terms with everything that happened was helped by firstly, going through my notes so that I could piece together what happened and most importantly, talking again and again about the section to Malcolm who was brilliant and coped marvellously although he says he was in a state of shock for a long time.*'

'*What helped me recover from the experience was joining a Caesarean Support Group. Helping other women get through the tough times helped me to heal my own hurt.*'

FEELINGS ABOUT YOUR BABY

SOME WOMEN'S feelings for their baby are immensely strong from the moment of birth: '*My love for my baby was so amazing that I wanted another baby right away! And my friend who came to see me in hospital says my first words were, "I'll have to do this again; it's fantastic!"*'

They have an immense need to protect the baby and keep him close at all times: '*I held him the whole time. I didn't want to put him in the cot at the hospital and the midwife said, "Oh, you need some rest now". And I watched her put him in the cot and going out of the door and I just picked him up again.*'

As adults, we know that some couples fall in love at first sight; the minute they clap eyes on each other, they are sure that they were made to be together. For others, falling in love is a process which takes many months and perhaps years. Relationships which start in either way can be entirely satisfactory, and the fact that you're not a 'love at first sight' person doesn't reflect badly on your personality. What applies to adult relationships applies equally to forming a bond with a new baby; some women are instantly in love with their babies and others find their love grows gradually:

'*I can honestly say I didn't want to take my baby home from hospital. I wanted to leave him there and then when I did take him home, I felt nothing for him at all and that lasted for about four or five weeks. Now I feel that I am having a passionate love affair with my baby.'*

'I'd expected a sudden rush when I saw her and it was more gradual than that. It was very powerful, but not there all at once.'

FEEDING YOUR BABY

YOU WILL PROBABLY feel that the most important aspect of mothering, at least in the first days and weeks of your baby's life, is feeding her properly. The choice whether to bottle-fed or breastfeed is a very personal one:

'I can't understand why anybody wants to breastfeed. I see the bottle as the symbol of women's liberation.'

'I remember feeling really proud of my little boy who was still being breastfed at six months old and thinking, "That's all me; I've done that. One cell, that's all my husband put in!"'

The success of either method will depend, in large measure, on how happy you are about your decision and how well supported you are in it.

Whichever way you feed your baby, there will inevitably be things you worry about. It naturally seems immensely important in those first few weeks to get the feeding right, and midwives and health visitors sometimes appear to assess the quality of your mothering according to how much weight your baby is putting on. If you decide to bottle-feed your baby, you will doubtless be anxious about sterilising the bottles and making up the feeds correctly. You may have been shown how to do this by the community midwife or by a midwife on the postnatal ward in the hospital. If you haven't, you can follow the instructions on the tin of formula milk or box of sterilising tablets and you won't go wrong. Breastfeeding is a different kind of learning process. It involves the baby finding out how he can get the milk from the breast as efficiently as possible and the mother finding out how she can feed her baby as comfortably as possible.

PUTTING YOUR BABY TO THE BREAST

- Make sure that you are sitting or lying in a comfortable position with your back well supported. Use plenty of cushions or pillows to bring the baby up to the level of your breasts
- Hold your baby close and turn her so that her chest is facing your chest
- Make sure that her head is in line with her body and not turned to one side
- Position your baby so that her upper lip is on a level with your nipple. You can stimulate your baby to open her mouth by rubbing her top lip against your nipple
- Once her mouth opens *wide*, move her quickly onto the breast
  (Remember that she is going to take a lot of the breast into her mouth and not just your nipple, so her mouth needs to be *really wide open*)
- Relax and enjoy the feed!

Have I got it right?

Check: Are your baby's lips curled back? (You may need a mirror to see or a friend to tell you.)

Check: If you can still see some areola (the coloured skin around your nipple), more should be showing above your baby's top lip than below her bottom lip.

Check: Does it hurt you when your baby feeds? If it does, take her off the breast by slipping your finger into the corner of her mouth, and start again. You may experience a *strong* sensation (rather than a *painful* one) when your baby first starts feeding, but this should disappear within 5 or 6 seconds.

Check: Does your baby's feeding action seem to be strong and rhythmic so that you can see her ears wiggling or the muscles in her temples moving? Your baby uses her tongue and lower jaw to do the work of suckling so if her cheeks are moving in and out, she's not feeding properly and you need to take her off the breast and reposition her with her mouth wider open.

The right way of breastfeeding

- The baby feeds from the breast and not from the nipple
- The baby feeds at the breast for as often and for as long as she wants to
- The baby feeds from the first breast until it is soft and empty and then from the second only if she wants to
- The baby needs nothing except breast milk – she doesn't need formula milk and she doesn't need water.

REMEMBER
The more often you feed your baby, the more milk you will make. Your baby knows exactly how often to feed

All these are normal!

- Your baby feeds eight or ten times a day
- Your milk looks yellow in the early days and then thin and watery later on
- Your baby likes to feed for a long time
  Your baby feeds very quickly
- Your baby has a dirty nappy at every feed
  Your baby has one dirty nappy a day
  Your baby has one dirty nappy a week.

LOOKING AFTER YOURSELF WHEN YOU ARE BREASTFEEDING

- Eat well and regularly. If you haven't time to make meals and haven't someone who can make them for you, have lots of healthy snacks such as sandwiches, cereal, nuts, raisins, fruit, yogurt

- Drink when you feel thirsty – water or fruit juice are ideal, but try and avoid drinks containing caffeine (coffee, tea, hot chocolate, cola) and having more than the odd glass of alcohol. You don't have to drink milk to make milk, but it can be a useful snack

- Rest as much as you can.

If you eat, drink and rest, you'll make plenty of milk for your baby and you'll enjoy feeding her.

Some babies just seem to get the hang of breastfeeding straight away, to the surprise of their mothers who had anticipated that it would be far more difficult than it turns out to be: *'I used to get sore painful breasts every month before my period, and I thought it would be like that when I fed, but it was much nicer.'*

But other women have to persevere and work their way through problems such as sore nipples and the anxiety of not knowing whether the baby has had enough milk before they reach the desired goal of effortless breastfeeding: *'I can't wait for the moment when I can just casually stick her on without having to think about it.'*

The first days are generally the most difficult and it's in this initial period that a lot of women sadly give up breastfeeding or come very close to it: *'I loved my baby, but there were times when I just wished I didn't have to be the one to feed her.'*

Tiredness can make the effort of acquiring a new skill seem too great, and the attractions of a different form of infant feeding very strong. However, not every woman who chooses to bottle-feed is

GETTING HELP WITH BREASTFEEDING

If you're worried about breastfeeding, or you have a problem such as your nipples getting sore, don't struggle on alone. You can get help from:

- Your midwife
- Your health visitor
- A breastfeeding counsellor
  - from The National Childbirth Trust
  - from La Leche League
  (You don't have to be a member of these organisations to contact one of their counsellors. Counsellors are there to give support and information to any woman who needs it.)

entirely without her depressed moments either: '*I was up to here with sterilising bottles.*'

Becoming more confident about your chosen method of feeding will go hand in hand with seeing your baby grow and develop: '*Only one thing kept me going: Jacob's obvious pleasure in breastfeeding and his bouncing good health.*'

If you find yourself the focus of conflicting advice about infant feeding, try to decide who are the people who make you feel good about your mothering and listen to them. People who undermine your confidence will be of no service to you at all; those who are supportive are the ones who will enable you to feel happy and be successful as a mother: '*Solomon was feeding all day and I was convinced that I didn't have enough milk. Fortunately, the midwife was still seeing me and she examined my breasts and said, "Nonsense, you could feed the street." It gave me a real boost of confidence.*'

LOOKING AFTER YOUR BABY

BECAUSE FAIRLY few women nowadays have looked after or even held a small baby before they give birth to their own, the day-to-day practicalities of caring for a new baby can be very daunting. A century ago, women had probably had experience of carrying out or at least observing babycare tasks from a very early age. Today, we have to learn how to care for our babies by reading books, asking other people and, ultimately, by having a go:

'*The first nappy change took half an hour and that was two of us, running up and down stairs because everything was in the wrong place. If anyone had had a video and could have filmed this little baby just lying there patiently while these two crazy people ran around the house . . . Well!*'

'*I just didn't feel confident about holding her. In the end, Orlando said, "Do you think she ought to have a bath today?" and we both did it together. It was like surgery. We laid out towels all over her bedroom floor and he fetched the bath and filled it with water and we'd got bubble bath and all the kits that people buy you and we really didn't use any of it. We just sort of plopped her in*' and plopped her out again and that was it. I was so worried that she'd get cold.'

With second babies, mothers find that they are far more relaxed, far less particular, and often far more able to enjoy the early weeks of their new child's life:

'Second babies are far easier than first. I made such hard work of it first time even though he was a very good baby. I did it all by the book; I was always washing. Everything took me so long.'

'She'd sleep for six hours and I'd wonder if there was something wrong – babies are not meant to sleep that long! Second time round, you're just happy to let them carry on sleeping.'

Eventually, first-time mothers too become more confident in themselves and more confident in their babies: 'You finally cotton on that you don't have to be so pedantic, that the baby will survive.'

LACK OF SLEEP

THE MAJORITY of parents are astonished to find how little rest they get during the first weeks of their babies' lives and how difficult it is to be constantly deprived of sleep. While most of us are used to having the odd sleepless night and the odd occasion when we don't get to bed at all, having no sleep for days on end puts people under a strain they may never have experienced before.

Some women find that they can be very philosophical about broken nights: 'I am surprised that I can keep going day and night because I'm a person who really likes my sleep. I'm surprised that if she cries in the night, I just think, "Oh, she's crying," and I'm quite happy to go to her. I'm not cross; it doesn't worry me that she's sometimes up all night and that surprises me.'

For others the long disturbed nights are very distressing: 'Elizabeth never let me sleep and I got so exhausted. It was quite a black period for a long time. I was just so tired.'

SLEEPLESS NIGHTS

- Help the baby to get into a routine by giving him minimum stimulation at night:
  - Don't change him unless he's obviously wet or dirty
    - Don't play with him
    - Keep the lighting low
    - Feed him and put him down again immediately.
- Discuss with your partner whether it would be a good idea for you to have separate rooms for a while so that only one person needs to be disturbed for night feeds
- Or share the night-time feeding and changing
- During the day, rest whenever and wherever you can
- Ask for help during the day so that you can rest
- Remember that the baby will develop a routine, but in his own time which could take a few months.

'I remember begging the baby for sleep — "Just five minutes, please give me five minutes." Two hours later, I was still begging him for five minutes.'

For the first few weeks of their lives, there are probably no babies who are 'in a routine' even though many parents want to encourage this at all costs. Routines are very helpful for small children and adults, but they have no relevance at all to babies: *'I just couldn't understand why my baby didn't sleep. She wouldn't go down until four in the morning, and then she would be awake at six or six thirty again for another feed. And she was unpredictable; she never slept at any set times. It is getting better.'*

Some women become experts at sleeping wherever and whenever the opportunity arises: *'In the night, I'm half sleeping anyway when I feed him and I can instantly go back to sleep when he's finished. Often if he sleeps during the day, I just stretch out on the couch with a book and fall asleep. I think you have to do that; it's the only way to keep going.'*

When you're adjusting to motherhood with your first baby, it can seem that the pattern of broken nights is a fixed one and that the baby will never sleep for more than two or three hours without requiring attention. In the vast majority of cases, however, babies do grow into the habit of sleeping for nine or ten hours at night-time without waking at all. It's important, if at all possible, to hang on to the comforting thought that your tiny, extremely demanding baby will grow into a little person who has come to grips with the difference between day and night: *'Remember that everything is a phase. Nothing lasts very long. However bad it is today, another couple of weeks down the line and everything will be different.'*

CRYING BABIES

IT IS SAID that most adults find the noise of a baby crying intolerable after only a few minutes. Parents become frantic when they can't stop their babies crying. A howling baby makes you feel very incompetent as a mother and there's always the worry at the back of your mind that there may be something seriously wrong. Nine times out of ten, the baby is crying because he is hungry, but there are occasions in every mother's life when she has fed her baby repeatedly, changed him, cuddled him, and done everything she can think of to soothe him and he still goes on crying:

'The baby's crying – you get the milk ready and tell him it's warming up. You give it to him. No, he's still crying, it wasn't that; it must be the nappy. You go upstairs and change the nappy. That doesn't work either – he's still crying. It probably means that he's too hot. You check him and put something cooler on; now he's crying because he's too cold. Perhaps it's wind – and by that time, you wonder if he's screaming because he's hungry again.'

Mothers can be driven to behave in ways they would never have imagined possible when their babies cry endlessly: *'One night, I rang for help at two o'clock in the morning, and the only midwife I could find said, "Will you harm your baby?" and I said, "I'm not going to harm the baby, but I can't stop him crying and I don't want him". She was very helpful, but if someone had told me that that would happen to me, I would never have believed them because I have loved babies for as long as I can remember.'*

WHEN THE BABY CRIES AND CRIES

- Try feeding her (again)
- Then try:
  - Changing her nappy
  - Checking that she is not too warm/too cold
  - Rocking her
  - Holding her
  - Singing to her
  - Playing music to her
  - Taking her for a drive in the car
- Get some support
  - Hand the baby over to your partner, grandparent, sister, relative, friend, next door neighbour and have a break
- If the baby is fed, clean and clearly not ill, put her in her cot, shut the door and retreat for a fixed period of time to a room where you cannot hear her crying. After – and only after – the fixed time has gone by, go and check her. With a bit of luck, she'll be fast asleep
- If you're at all worried about the baby's health, call the doctor
- Contact CRY-SIS or another parents' organisation and talk to someone who understands what you are going through
- Remember that it's OK to feel angry and frustrated sometimes; life with a baby is hard work.

It's quite common for babies to have periods of crying and restlessness in the early hours of the evening. The mother is tired at the end of her day and perhaps her tiredness and stress transmit themselves to the baby. Often it's impossible to find out why the baby is upset and once you have grown a little in confidence, you come to accept it as one of those things:

'Usually from 7.30 in the evening through till 9.30, she cries. It seems to be her crying time. After several attempts to put her down, she gets to the point where she just goes off.'

'He's obviously exhausted, absolutely exhausted, but he won't go in his cot. He's crying because he's so tired but he just wants to be among us.'

Women are often aware that the more uptight they are, the more fretful the baby becomes; trying to relax can be the answer – but that's often easier said than done! If it's possible to hand the baby over to someone else when you're exhausted with trying to soothe him, then don't hesitate to do so. Learning to ask for and to accept help is not easy for many women, but the more support you can get during the early days, months and years of motherhood, the more likely you are to enjoy them: *'If people offer to help, then accept it. I should have done that. I was a real martyr. I'd say, "It's okay, I can manage. I can do ten things at once!" And you can't really. Inside, you're quivering.'*

BEING A MOTHER

SOME WOMEN seem to love being a mother from the word 'go' and have no difficulties in adjusting: *'It's wonderful and a lot easier than I expected.'*

It's probably more common to find that getting used to your new role takes time. Having a first baby may show you aspects of your personality which you were never aware of before. It can be very uncomfortable to find that you're not exactly the sort of person you thought you were: *'I used to work in a nursery for thirty children, and so I thought I would just sail through looking after my own baby. But after a few days of*

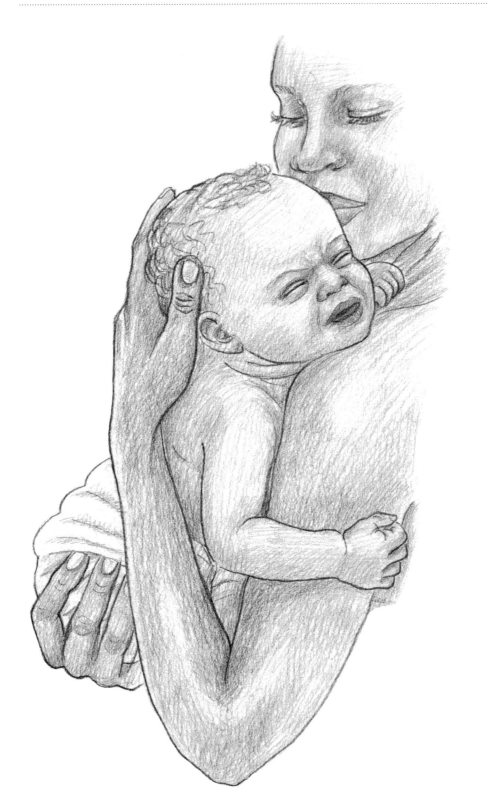

her constantly crying, I found I was running out of patience and I still do feel like that because she does cry a lot. I get cross with myself for being cross.'

Realising just how demanding motherhood is can be a shock:

'It's a tie that you've never had before so that even if you just want to hang washing on the line you have to think, "Where's the baby? What shall do I do with her? Will I take her with me or what?"'

'I want to take a shower without having to peep through the curtains and sing all the time just to try and calm this screaming infant down.'

Gradually, women are able to understand their own feelings better and to identify what they need if they are to be happy and effective as mothers:

'I get very frustrated. I need time with my partner, or with my friends, but definitely away from the baby.'

'The great day came when somebody offered to look after the baby for me. I was out of the door so fast and the first five minutes of freedom were marvellous.'

Along with a better understanding of their own needs, they also grow in confidence about looking after their babies and can decide for themselves what advice to accept and what to reject:

'They kept telling me to put the baby down. It finally clicked with me that I simply didn't agree with them. So I hardly put her down until she was crawling. That's what I wanted to do.'

Informed choices

'*That's what* I *wanted to do*' is the quotation which really sums up the theme of this book. Enjoying the experience of being pregnant, of giving birth to a baby and of becoming a mother is all about making your own decisions – after listening to the opinions of health professionals and other parents – but finally deciding for yourself what you want to do. You can learn from the experience and knowledge of others, but you then have to apply what they say to your own situation, and you are the expert about that. Your baby is uniquely yours; you know more about him than anyone else and your instinct as to what he needs and what you need in order to look after him is almost certainly going to be your best guide to making you both happy.

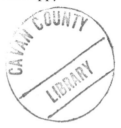

Useful Addresses

Making Decisions about Antenatal Testing

Harris Birthright Research Centre
King's College Hospital, Denmark Hill,
London SE5 8RX
Tel: 0171 924 0894/0714

St Bartholomew's Hospital Medical
College Antenatal Screening Service
Charterhouse Square,
London EC1M 6BQ
Tel: 0171 982 6293/4

Support After Termination for Fetal
Abnormality
(SATFA)
73 Charlotte Street
London W1P 1LB
Tel: 0171 631 0285

University of Leeds Down's Syndrome
Screening Service
Institute of Epidemiology,
34 Hyde Terrace,
Leeds LS2 9LN
Tel: 0113 234 4013

Babies and Children with Special Needs

Contact-a-Family
170 Tottenham Court Road
London W1P 0HA
Tel: 0171 383 3555
(Provides support and information for
families caring for children with any type
of disability or special need.)

The Association for Spina Bifida and
Hydrocephalus
ASBAH House, 42 Park Road,
Peterborough PE1 2UQ
Tel: 01733 555988

The Down's Syndrome Association
155 Mitcham Road,
London SW17 9PG
Tel: 0181 682 4001

Help if You are Using Illegal Drugs

Drugline
9A Brockley Cross, Brockley,
London SE4 2AB
Tel: 0181 692 4975

Contacting an Independent Midwife

Write to:
Lesley Hobbs
Independent Midwives Association
The Wessex Maternity Centre,
Mansbridge Road, West End,
Southampton SO18 3HW

Enclose an A5 stamped addressed envelope and you will be sent a register of all the independent midwives in the UK.

Employing a Doula

Birth and Bonding International
60 Nottingham Road,
Belper DE56 1JH
Tel: 01773 826055
(This organisation will be able to give you a list of doulas)

Hiring a Birthing Pool

Splashdown
17 Wellington Terrace
Harrow-on-the-Hill, London HA1 3EP
Tel: 0181 422 9308

Active Birth Centre
25 Bickerton Road, London N19 5JT
Tel: 0171 561 9006

Elsie Inglis Birth Pool,
40 Leamington Terrace
Edinburgh EH10 4JI
Tel: 0131 229 6259

Waterbabies
874 Burnley Road,
Walmersley, Bury,
Lancs BL9 5JY
Tel: 0161 764 2616

If You Need Support After a Caesarean

Contact:
The National Childbirth Trust
Alexandra House, Oldham Terrace,
Acton, London W3 6NH
Tel: 0181 992 8637

If Your Baby is in Special Care

Baby Life Support Systems
BLISS/NIPPERS
17–21 Emerald Street,
London WC1N 3QL
Tel: 0171 831 9393

The National Childbirth Trust
Alexandra House, Oldham Terrace,
Acton, London W3 6NH
Tel: 0181 992 8637

If you contact the headquarters of these organisations at the numbers given above, you will be told how to get in touch with someone close to where you live who can help you.

Hiring a Breast Pump

The National Childbirth Trust
Alexandra House, Oldham Terrace,
Acton, London W3 6NH
Tel: 0181 992 8637

La Leche League
BM3424, London WC1N 3XX
Tel: 0171 242 1278

The cost is approximately 85p per day plus an initial £8.50 which you pay for the milk collection set. Both these organisations can generally offer a reduced fee if this is too much for you to pay.

If Your Baby Dies

Compassionate Friends
53 North Street, Bristol BS3 1EN
Tel: 0117 966 5202
Helpline: Monday-Friday, 9.30am–5pm:
0117 953 9639

Stillbirth and Neonatal Death Society
(SANDS)
28 Portland Place,
London W1N 4DE
Tel: 0171 436 5881

Miscarriage Association
c/o Clayton Hospital
Northgate, Wakefield
West Yorkshire WF1 3JS
Tel: 01924 200799

If Your Baby Cries a Lot

CRY-SIS
BM Cry-sis,
London WC1N 3XX
Tel: 0171 404 5011

National Association of Parents of
Sleepless Children
PO Box 33,
Prestwood, Gt Missenden,
Bucks NH16 0SZ
No telephone number

Meeting Other Mums

Meet-A-Mum-Association
14 Willis Road,
Croydon
Surrey CR2O 2XX
Tel: 0181 665 0357
Fax: 0181 665 1972
Helpline 3pm–11pm: 0181 656 7318

The National Childbirth Trust
Alexandra House, Oldham Terrace,
Acton, London W3 6NH
Tel: 0181 992 8637

Index